MODERN CHINA AND TRADITIONAL CHINESE MEDICINE

MODERN CHINA
AND TRADITIONAL
CHINESE MEDICINE

A Symposium Held at the
University of Wisconsin, Madison

Edited by

GUENTER B. RISSE, M.D., Ph.D.

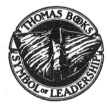

CHARLES C THOMAS · PUBLISHER

Springfield · Illinois · U.S.A.

CHARLES C THOMAS • PUBLISHER
Springfield • Illinois • U.S.A.
Published and Distributed Throughout the World by
CHARLES C THOMAS • PUBLISHER
Bannerstone House
301-327 East Lawrence Avenue, Springfield, Illinois, U.S.A.

©*1973, by* CHARLES C THOMAS • PUBLISHER
ISBN 0-398-02816-8
Library of Congress Catalog Card Number: 73-201

*With THOMAS BOOKS careful attention is given to all details of
manufacturing and design. It is the Publisher's desire to present books that are
satisfactory as to their physical qualities and artistic possibilities and
appropriate for their particular use. THOMAS BOOKS will be true to those
laws of quality that assure a good name and good will.*

32113

Printed in the United States of America
I-1

PARTICIPANTS

JAMES Y. P. CHEN, M.D.
Staff Physician
Southern California Edison Co.
Los Angeles, California

RALPH C. CROIZIER, PH.D.
Associate Professor
Department of History
University of Rochester
Rochester, New York

KENNETH LEVIN
Ph.D. Candidate in Modern Chinese History
University of Wisconsin
Visiting Instructor
Department of History
Antioch College
Yellow Springs, Ohio

PAUL PICKOWICZ
Ph.D. Candidate in Modern Chinese History
University of Wisconsin
Fellow, East Asian Research Center,
Harvard University
Cambridge, Massachusetts

GUENTER B. RISSE, M.D., PH.D.
Associate Professor and Chairman
Department of the History of Medicine
University of Wisconsin Center for
*   Health Sciences*
Madison, Wisconsin

SAMUEL ROSEN, M.D.
Clinical Professor of Otology
Mt. Sinai School of Medicine of the
*   City of New York*

Consulting Ear Surgeon
New York Eye and Ear Infirmary
New York, New York

C. NORMAN SHEALY, M.D.
Director
Pain Rehabilitation Center
La Crosse, Wisconsin

ILZA VEITH, PH.D.
Professor and Vice-Chairman
Department of the History of Health Sciences
University of California
San Francisco, California

NANCY N. WU, M.D.
Assistant Professor
Department of Anesthesiology
University of Wisconsin
Center for Health Sciences
Madison, Wisconsin

CONTENTS

vii

MODERN CHINA AND TRADITIONAL CHINESE MEDICINE

PART I
(INTRODUCTION)

> Unite all medical workers, young and old, of the traditional school and modern school, and organize a solid united front to strive for the development of the people's health.
>
> — Mao Tse-tung

IN PLANNING THIS SYMPOSIUM for April 15, 1972, on the eve of the 25th anniversary of the creation of a chair in medical history at the University of Wisconsin, it was my desire to furnish a forum for the scholarly discussion of Chinese medicine. Such a timely subject has recently received wide diffusion throughout the country both in newspapers and popular magazines. Over two decades of pent-up curiosity and an old fascination with the Orient have made us thirsty for new knowledge concerning an old civilization.

With the thaw in Chinese-American relations begun by the so-called "ping-pong diplomacy" of last year, two American scientists visited the People's Republic in May 1971: Arthur W. Galston, a molecular biologist from Yale University, and Ethan Signer, a plant physiologist from M.I.T. Both were the first American men of science to visit mainland China since 1949. After spending about two weeks in that country, they returned to the U.S. with strange-sounding accounts about the use of traditional Chinese acupuncture as the sole anesthetic agent in a variety of surgical procedures.

As it turned out, both Galston and Signer had requested from their hosts a visit to a Chinese hospital in order to acquire an impression of the present status of their medicine. Their wishes were granted, and to the surprise of the American visitors, they witnessed a series of operations with conventional and electro-acupuncture at one of the hospitals affiliated with Peking Medical College. Unsurprisingly, upon their return both scientists encountered great skepticism and mainly disbelief about their stories.

Then, last September, the Bamboo Curtain opened even

5

further to allow the entrance of four distinguished American physicians, the first ones to visit China in twenty-two years. The group was composed of Drs. E. Grey Dimond, a cardiologist and provost for Health Sciences at the University of Missouri, Victor W. Sidel, Chief of the Department of Social Medicine, Montefiore Hospital in the Bronx, Paul Dudley White, distinguished Boston cardiologist and Samuel Rosen, the noted otolaryngologist and pioneer of the stapes mobilization procedure for deafness. All four physicians traveled through China with their wives for several weeks, and upon their return confirmed the previous reports about acupuncture anesthesia. Moreover, they were greatly impressed about the impact which the various and successful public campaigns were having on the health of the Chinese people, as, for example, the erradication of venereal diseases.

Again, as with Galston's previous accounts, these impressions gathered by the American physicians received wide press coverage in this country. A medically oriented report on both acupuncture and modern Chinese medical education by Dr. Dimond was published late last year in the *Journal of the American Medical Association.* Although some physicians seemed impressed, others considered the reports a "hearsay, hear-see Marco Polo story," talking about hypnotic suggestions and naked political pressure as the factors responsible for the array of incomprehensible events described by the recent medical visitors.

As mentioned earlier, newspaper reporters and other non-medical witnesses have now had their say in a variety of popular publications concerning the subject of Chinese medicine. These accounts have largely accomplished their initial purpose of drawing our attention to the medical conditions and practices presently in existence in the People's Republic of China. I feel, like others, that it is now time to settle down for the more serious task of examining critically and scientifically the medical claims and accomplishments of a society which is politically and culturally quite alien to our own.

Thus, the purpose of the symposium was to bring together a group of scholars representing a variety of fields such as

Chinese history, anesthesiology, neurophysiology and medical history in an effort to clarify certain issues. More important, however, was the expectation that new questions and approaches would emerge from such an interdisciplinary setting. It is obvious that we cannot leave the entire subject matter in a sort of Marco Polo fairyland susceptible to ridicule and even contempt. By the same token, it is not possible to uncritically accept all travelers' accounts in spite of the enthusiasm and good faith of those who were privileged to recently visit China.

I believe that the time has come for initiating a sober and dispassionate evaluation of the recent developments in medicine and public health which have taken place in the People's Republic of China. Instead of dismissing the events as charlatanism, mass hypnosis or political indoctrination, we must wrestle with the new facts and subject them to serious scientific scrutiny. Too much is at stake for us, especially in the fields of health care delivery, public and community health and anesthesiology.

If we maintain a narrow and parochial viewpoint and refuse to use our scientific resources for the study of Chinese medicine, the entire field will fall into the hands of less well-trained opportunists. With their bizarre claims and cloak of mystery these individuals will only contribute to a total discredit and rejection of a medical system which indeed may offer valuable lessons for the West. To date only a selected few Americans have been able to travel to the People's Republic of China. Three participants of our symposium have done so within the last year and their valuable and interesting experiences have been collected here.

Thus, my primary reason for publishing the proceedings of the symposium has been to make this information available to the reader interested in the subject of Chinese medicine. This book should only be viewed as an interim document which modestly hopes to somewhat fill the gap of our knowledge about Chinese medicine until more American scholars can visit mainland China and furnish us with more extensive and precise data. In the midst of a veritable flood of popular writings, the proceedings of this symposium will give the discriminating reader a more sober and scholarly source of information. A glance at the table of contents will reveal that the topic of acupuncture has received more attention and merited more articles than any other subject. This fact in no way implies that other Chinese accomplishments in the field of health care delivery have been neglected or ignored. However, the present wave of sensationalism surrounding acupuncture prompted me to furnish the reader with a sobering and scholarly array of articles which places this healing method in a better perspective.

All our speakers at the Symposium have kindly consented to expand their remarks and have included bibliographical references. In addition, I have included two original Chinese reports and added a general bibliography which may aid the reader interested in enlarging his knowledge about China and its medicine.

The theme for the entire book was coined by Professor Croizier as being one of "suspended judgment." The articles are largely descriptive in character and only in certain instances has it been possible to make tentative interpretations. While the jury is still out such a collection of facts must continue through further exchanges of information and scholars between our two countries.

Beyond a selfish and utilitarian reason for studying events which could benefit our own teaching and practice of medicine, there is another dimension. The Canadian physician Dr. Wilder Penfield, one of the world's foremost neurosurgeons and neurologists, eloquently expressed this aspect after his return from the People's Republic of China in 1962: "The time has come for an offensive of friendship. The house of world peace will never be built until and unless its foundation is laid in the understanding that men were born to be brothers — all men." Therefore, as the Bamboo Curtain hopefully rises in the months and years ahead, let us approach one-fourth of mankind in that spirit of understanding and brotherhood.

Guenter B. Risse

REFERENCES

Dimond, E.G.: "Acupuncture anesthesia: Western medicine and Chinese traditional medicine," *J.A.M.A.* 218 (1971), 1558-1563.

Galston, A.W.: "Attitudes on acupuncture 1971," *The Yale Review* 61 (1971), 312-317.

Penfield, W.: "Oriental renaissance in education and medicine." *Science* 141 (1963), 1153-1161.

Penfield, Wilder: *The Chinese People's Republic: A Physician's Observations*, Horowitz Lectures 1963, New York, Inst. Phys. Med. & Rehab. N.Y.U., 1963. (Rehabilitation Monograph XXIII)

Rosen, S.: "I have seen the past and it works," *New York Times*, November 1st and November 4, 1971.

Signer, E. and Galston, A.W.: "Education and science in China," *Science* 175 (1972), 15-23.

White, P.D.: "China's heart is in the right place," *New York Times*, December 5, 1971.

PART II
(HISTORICAL BACKGROUND)

Chapter 1

TRADITIONAL CHINESE MEDICINE: HISTORICAL REVIEW

Ilza Veith

W ITH THE RESUMPTION OF POLITICAL, diplomatic, scientific, and cultural relations between the United States and China a veritable epidemic of interest has developed in America in the seemingly most bizarre aspect of Chinese medicine. Apparently the American visitors to China believed they had "discovered" acupuncture as though it were an entirely new phenomenon in the long history of Chinese medicine.

Indeed, the American visitors, no matter whether they were diplomats, "China Scholars," ping-pong players, or even physicians, were so overwhelmed by the dramatic use of acupuncture anesthesia in major surgery that they failed to realize that this was the only *new* aspect of acupuncture, whereas, in fact, the practice of needling dates back at least seven thousand years to Neolithic times when the first needles were made of stone.

Thus acupuncture is only a part of a rich, intricate, and ancient medical system which must be appreciated in its totality in order to yield an explanation for the phenomena that were observed by the recent American visitors.

The origins of China's medical history are veiled in legend. Tradition ascribes the oldest Chinese medical work, the *Huang Ti Nei Ching Su Wen "The Yellow Emperor's Classic of Internal Medicine,"* to the authorship of Huang Ti, the Yellow Emperor, whose life span is said to have extended from 2697 to 2597 B.C.

While it is not possible to state with any certainty when this great work was actually written down, a number of textual references and many touches of Taoist thinking point to the 4th or 3rd century B.C. The form in which *The Yellow Emperor's Classic of Internal Medicine* has come down to us was given to it in 762 A.D. by Wang Ping of the Tang dynasty, the ablest and most vigorous of the many scholars who interpreted, commented upon, and elaborated this fundamental book, which is even now the basis of Chinese medicine.

It is significant in many ways that the work should have been attributed to an emperor traditionally accorded such an early rule. Even at the time when it was first conceived, the *Classic* was obviously destined to be of lasting value, and its actual author, or authors, sacrificed the desire for personal glory to the supreme task of creating a work for eternity. This could best be done by ascribing the authorship to an exalted and ancient being, for China's reverence of antiquity dates back to its earliest days.

The naming of one of the ancients as an author was not without some justification, since the wording of the work makes it evident that its contents had been the intellectual property of the Chinese for a very long time before they were formulated and put down. The traditional dates of Huang Ti, the Yellow Emperor, make him a perfect choice for the hypothetical author of a work that stresses health and long life. He himself is supposed to have lived for one entire century and this, according to the *Classic*, is the ideal span of life. But there is another, and perhaps the most interesting, purpose which can be inferred from the title of the *Yellow Emperor's Classic of Internal Medicine*, and even more from the form of the text itself: the work is written in the form of a dialogue between Huang Ti and his Prime Minister Ch'i Po, in which the Emperor — often in the humblest way — seeks instruction in all questions pertaining to health and the art of healing.

Although this conversation can hardly be considered a historical fact, the involvement of the names of these two personages is strongly indicative of the exalted place accorded to medicine in ancient China. It seems certain that the authors of the *Classic* considered knowledge of the forces that cause life and death worthy of an Emperor and the art of healing to be the predominant responsibility of the elect. The grave obligation imposed by the mastery of the healing art finds expression in the Emperor's solemn vow: "I shall smear my mouth with blood and take an oath that I will not venture to receive this information were I to use it recklessly or neglect it."

Beyond doubt, the practice of medicine has often been connected with an awareness of the moral responsibilities of the practitioner, and the wording of the Yellow Emperor's vow brings to mind the Hippocratic Oath. But the *Huang Ti Nei Ching Su Wen* differs from the Hippocratic writings which form the basis of Western medicine. The latter were written to give practical advice to the practicing physician; the former goes far beyond the scope of a medical text-book, being a treatise on life itself.

In the modern mind medicine is regarded as perhaps the most highly developed of all natural sciences. Religion, philosophy, thoughts on cosmogony and the course of the universe hardly influence the actions of the present-day physician; ethics is a professional guide that helps the doctor guard himself from professional mistakes, and perhaps against malpractice suits, but the patient's ethics, except in so far as it may influence his psychological well-being, is of no concern to the physician.

The immense difference in the ancient Chinese concept of the art of healing can best be illustrated by a short passage from the *Classic*:

[The Yellow Emperor said] "I urge you to bring into harmony for me nature, Heaven, and Tao [the right way]. There must be an end and a beginning. Heaven must be in accord with the lights of the sky, the celestial bodies, and their course and periods. The earth below must reflect the four seasons, the five elements, that which is precious and that which is lowly and without value—one as well as the other. Is it not that in Winter man responds to Yin [the principle of darkness and cold]? And is it not that in Summer he responds to Yang [the principle of light and warmth]? Let me be informed about their workings."

Ch'i Po replied: "Truly a subtle question! It demands that one decipher Nature to the utmost degree."

The Emperor exclaimed: "I should like to be informed about Nature to the utmost degree and include (information) about man, his physical form, his blood, his breath of life, his flowing and his dissolution; and I should like to know what causes his death and his life and what we can do about all this."

Here we see the essence of early Chinese medical thinking. A medical science did not exist by itself, the art of healing was part of philosophy and religion, both of which propounded oneness with nature and the universe.

The *Yellow Emperor's Classic* was written long after theories of cosmogony and the workings of the universe had been conceived and become formalized. The work does not contain basic explanations of phenomena, since the reader was expected to be familiar with the most important concepts of philosophy and religion. Before these concepts are explained here, it must be stated that there was little or no distinction between religious and philosophical thought in ancient China. Nor does the word religion in this context refer to any of the three major cults: Confucianism, Taoism and Buddhism. To be sure, certain elements of Confucian and Taoist doctrine can be found in the philosophic-religious thought of the *Classic,* but they are representative of the earlier writings rather than of the later, formalized cults.

In the passage of the *Classic* quoted above, mention is made of the three essential features which form the basis of all reasoning underlying Chinese Universalism in general, the *Huang Ti Nei Ching Su Wen* in particular, and finally Chinese medical thinking in its entirety. These three features are the *Tao,* the *Yin* and the *Yang,* and the 5 elements, all of which have their place and function in the Chinese concept of the creation of the world. Since Chinese traditional thinking conceives of man as composed of the same elements as the universe and as functioning along the same principles as the macrocosm, it might be well here to summarize briefly the Chinese concept of cosmogony.

That this concept was the result of philosophical rather than religious thinking becomes immediately evident when one realizes that creation was never attributed to a superior or superhuman being. It was thought that the world had created itself, driven by Tao, an abstract motivator, which remained active and turned into a moral guide, once creation was accomplished. It was Tao, the Way, that caused the original state of chaos to divide into two forces, known as the Yin and the Yang, the female and the male, the negative and the positive elements. Even after creation was completed, Tao remained effective in guiding the functions of everything within the universe, while Yin and Yang in their ebb and flow of opposition and attraction to each other maintained all things and beings of the newly created world in their proper balance and harmony.

During creation, the Yin and the Yang brought forth the 5 elements: water, fire, wood, metal and earth. These formed the material substance for everything in this world. The correct proportion of these elements was preserved by the workings of the Tao and the interaction of the Yin and Yang.

In the macrocosm the visible results of perfect balance were the change from day to night, the rising and the setting of the sun, the waxing and the waning of the moon, the unchangeable sequences of the seasons, the planting and the growing of the crops. Droughts and floods, failure of the crops and other natural phenomena were indications of a disturbance in the balance of nature.

Man, who was created with the universe and in its image, owed his health and hence his life to the harmony of natural forces; if this harmony was upset, the result was disease and death. But while the macrocosm of the universe was left to the course of Tao and the natural forces, it was up to man to shape his fate by compliance with Tao, the Way, and thus to keep the proper balance of Yin and Yang, the two opposing forces.

The Yellow Emperor's Classic is the first book that explains to man what he can expect by living according to the Tao and thus according to nature, and how he can learn to adapt his life to this system:

> Just as the breath of the blue sky (is calm), so the will and the heart of those who are pure will be in peace, and the breath of Yang will be stable in those who keep themselves in harmony with nature. Even if there are noxious spirits they cannot cause injury to those who follow the laws of the seasons.

But the book also stresses the effects of disobedience to the Tao, the resulting disease and premature deterioration:

> Those who fail to preserve this (good conduct) will have their nine orifices closed from the inside, and the development of their muscles and flesh will be obstructed from the outside, and the breath of protection will be lost to them. This then is called: "to injure one's own body and to destroy one's own force of life."

The preceding quotations show that the *Classic* was directed to the educated layman as well as to the physician, but for the latter it has much specific advice which reaches its highest wisdom in the following exhortation:

> . . . the sages did not treat those who were already ill; they instructed those who were not yet ill. They did not want to rule those who were already rebellious; they guided those who were not yet rebellious. To administer medicines to diseases which have already developed and to suppress revolts which have already developed is comparable to the behaviour of those persons who begin to dig a well after they have become thirsty, and of those who begin to cast weapons after they have already engaged in battle. Would these actions not be too late?

It is easy to see why the Chinese conceived a naturalistic philosophy and clung to it for thousands of years. They have been and still are to a large extent an agricultural people, totally dependent upon nature's immutable course. Thus it was natural for them to think of themselves as one with the universe which provided them so directly with their livelihood. Because of this it was possible for the theories of *The Yellow Emperor's Classic* to become the basis of all subsequent medical writings and to survive up to the present day.

One may wonder how this transfer of the concepts of the macrocosm to the body of the human being was brought about. First of all, it must be said that this could have taken place only in a society that venerated the ancestor — and hence the dead — that considered the study of anatomy a desecration of the dead, and the performance of surgery a permanent disfigurement and an infringement upon the sacredness of the body. In such an atmosphere of thought, the human structure and the physiological processes could not be investigated; they had to be taken for granted. It will be realized that under these conditions it was possible to explain human anatomy and physiology by an analogy to the universe and in terms of the theories of Tao, Yin and Yang and the 5 elements. The following discussion will reveal that such analogies were not carried out altogether arbitrarily, and that occasional flashes of insight and wisdom went into their

ling taboos, *The Yellow Emperor's* Chinese medical works restricted ᴊ to a vague study of surface anato- che exterior of the body consisted of ᴊdons and bones. In addition there were ᴊed by the eyes, the nose, the mouth, the ᴊral openings. The description of internal ᴊs was as follows: man was composed of *Tsang*, or storing organs, and the 6 *Fu*, or The 5 *Tsang*, which were held to be more eliminating organs, were the liver, the heart, ᴊ, the kidneys. The 6 *Fu* were the stomach, he small intestine, the urinary bladder, the he "three burning spaces" — an imaginary components were held to be distributed over nd lower parts of the body. The storing and eliminating organs were connected by a system of vessels of which there were two kinds: those which carried blood and those which carried air or a vital pneuma.

This is a bare outline of the existing anatomical descriptions, but it may be sufficient to establish a parallel with the components of the universe and to form a basis for theories on the functions of the organs. In the *Classic* the Yellow Emperor is quoted as saying:

> Covered by Heaven and supported by Earth, all creation together in its most complete perfection is planned for the greatest achievement: Man. Man lives on the breath of Heaven and Earth and he achieves perfection through the laws of the four seasons.

The analogy between the human being and the 4 seasons was fortified by a preconceived numerical concept of the components of man: thus the body was believed to consist of 365 individual parts obviously corresponding with the 365 days of the year; the number of main vessels or meridians that carried blood and air was 12 and thus conformed with the 12 months; and lastly there were the *Tsang*, the 5 main organs representing the 5 elements.

Physiology, like anatomy, was based on the theories governing the creation of the world. The functioning of the body depended upon the two forces that created the world and men, the Yin and the Yang. While Yang, the male or positive principle, predominated in man, and Yin, the female or negative principle, predominated in woman, neither of these forces ever existed alone, but a certain proportion of both had to be present in every well-functioning human being. These two ever-active forces, alternately opposing and supplementing each other, were held to exist within all parts of the body and to circulate through the vessels that carried blood and pneuma. Pathological conditions arose out of abundance of either the Yin or the Yang, obstruction of the flow of blood and especially the pneuma. All these deficiencies and obstructions disturbed the balance of the organism as a whole, but usually affected one particular organ.

The concept of a disease entity as it is known to modern medicine did not exist in traditional Chinese thought. Some specific fevers were known and even distinguished according to a vague groping toward a knowledge of etiology, but even the possible causes of disease were subordinated to the general scheme of the universe. Thus, the 5 atmospheric conditions — wind, heat, humidity, dryness and cold — closely related to the 5 elements, could bring about such diseases as "injuries of the cold" (this group included typhoid fever,) "injuries of the heat," "the wind within," "humid warmth," etc. Smallpox, leprosy and various forms of intermittent fevers were also believed to arise out of atmospheric conditions. But it was generally believed that whatever immediate cause was held to be responsible for a particular disease, the patient had laid himself open to such an attack by a major infringement of Tao, the Way, and the invariable result was a disturbance of the balance of Yin and Yang.

It is noteworthy that *The Yellow Emperor's Classic* does not present these doctrines in flat statements, but that they are clothed in symbolic imagery which compare the functioning of the body to that of a state. The relations of the various organs to each other are likened to those of the high officials, and all are dependent upon the heart, which is described as "the minister of the monarch who excels through insight and understanding." It may well be that the following paragraphs were meant to carry a political as well as a medical message, although the text is presumably concerned with the body:

> When the monarch is intelligent and enlightened, there is peace and contentment among his subjects; they can thus beget offspring, and bring up their children, earn a living and lead a long and happy life.

> But when the monarch is not intelligent and enlightened, the twelve officials (the organs of the body) become dangerous and perilous; the use of Tao (the Right Way), is obstructed and blocked, and Tao no longer circulates warnings against physical excesses.

> Afflicted are those who dissipate; they become nervous and startled. But those who are aware of their needs and desires are encouraged, and as an expression of this encouragement they become peace-loving and virtuous.

By means of these apparent theories, the ancient Chinese arrived at two extremely important conclusions: first, that disease is rarely localized, but generally affects the entire human being; and, secondly, that disease is often associated with behaviour and with a feeling of guilt, derived from the infringement of a moral law. *The Yellow Emperor's Classic* abounds in statements concerning the effect of emotional states on health which can truly be termed precursors of psychosomatic medicine. It might be well here to quote some of the most pertinent ones:

> The Yellow Emperor said; "Man's place of residence, his motion and rest (his circumstances of life), his courage and cowardice—do they not also cause change within the vascular system (pulse)?"

> Ch'i Po answered: "Yes, in general, man's fear and apprehension, his passion (anger) and his suffering, his motion and his rest, they all cause changes."

"Therefore it is said: In order to examine the course of a disease one must investigate whether man is courageous or nervous and cowardly, and one must examine his bones, flesh, and skin and then one can know the facts which are necessary for the methods of treatment."

From the preceding discussion it is not to be wondered at that even the infringements of the laws of behaviour were systematized to the point of absurdity as may be seen in the following sentences:

Those whose demeanour is dissolute and licentious get a disease of the lungs. Those who are lazy and full of apprehension and fear, have difficulties in breathing, emanating from the lungs. Those whose demeanour is immoral and dissolute will injure their hearts.

Thus in Spring and in Fall, in Winter and in Summer, during the four seasons and during the periods of Yin and Yang, diseases are created, that are caused by faulty practices and transgressions which have become habit.

But even these schematizations do not detract from the basic wisdom which realized the existence of such a strong bond between the human body and the mind. With such principles in mind the ancient Chinese physician functioned not only as a healer of disease, but even more as a moral guide who helped his patient to acknowledge and rectify their infringements of moral and natural laws. Being a judge of man's behaviour as well as of his health presupposed a high moral and ethical attitude on the part of the early Chinese physician and a fairly well-organized state of the medical profession. And indeed, in the *Chou Li*, the "Rites of the Chou," whose dynasty flourished between 1122 and 221 B.C., we find the outlines of a medical organization with a well-defined hierarchy graded according to achievement and therapeutic success.

It is clear that neither the knowledge of disease as affecting the entire human being, nor the realization of a psychic factor as a cause, absolved the Chinese doctor from making a diagnosis of the nature and location of any particular illness. It is in the field of diagnosis that we find the least trace of realism and the greatest amount of schematization.

The main diagnostic method employed by the Chinese physician of antiquity, and still that of the traditional Chinese physician of today, is the taking of the pulse. This means of diagnosis is so intricate that it required several chapters in *The Yellow Emperor's Classic,* which were elaborated and expanded by Wang Shu-ho (about 280 A.D.) into a separate treatise of 10 volumes, entirely given over to the study of the pulse. The importance attributed throughout the centuries to pulse diagnosis can be gauged by the fact that from the time of Wang Shu-ho until today at least 156 additional books have appeared on the subject. The instructions concerning the pulse contained in *The Yellow Emperor's Classic* are briefly summarized here.

The pulse, it was said, consisted of 6 pulses on each wrist, each connected with a particular organ of the body, and each able to record even the minutest pathological changes taking place within the body. The procedure of palpation differed according to the sex of the patient; the physician first examined the pulses of the right wrist of female patients and those of the left wrist of male patients. By means of the pulse the physician was supposed to be able to judge the site and the state of the disease, its cause and duration, whether it was chronic or acute, and whether it would result in recovery or death. When we realize that the seasons, the time of day, weather conditions, and the age of the patient were held to cause differences in the sounds of the pulse beats, we become aware of the immense difficulties confronting the Chinese physician. And yet, their diagnoses were surprisingly accurate. Dr. Edward H. Hume, who was present at a number of such examinations, tells us that "many visits to patients in company with proficient Chinese physicians of the old school have shown . . . how almost uncanny is their power of recognition of organic conditions through pulse observation alone." Dr. Hume's statement finds corroboration from many other Western physicians who were astounded by the same phenomenon. A few selections from *The Yellow Emperor's Classic* may serve to illustrate the preceding discussions:

> The way of medical treatment is to be consistent. It should be executed at dawn when the breath of Yin has not yet begun to stir

and when the breath of Yang has not yet begun to diffuse; when food and drink have not yet been taken . . . when vigour and energy are not yet disturbed—at that particular time one should examine what has happened to the pulse.

If it were not for the excellent technique and the subtlety of the pulse one would not be able to examine it. But examination must be done according to plan and the system of Yin and Yang serve as basis for examination. When this basis is established, one can investigate the twelve main vessels and the five elements that generate life. Life itself follows a pattern that was set by the four seasons.

Those warm and genial days of Spring lead up to heat of Summer, and the anger one might feel in Autumn makes way for forgiveness and mercy which one feels in Winter. This change of the four seasons influences the upper and the lower pulses.

Diagnosis of the pulse was supplemented by a study of the patient's complexion, the changes of which were held to be indicative of the future development of the disease. The examination of the colours of the various parts of the body was carried out according to a fixed system of correlations between colours and "intestines" rather than according to actually observable phenomena. The ancient Chinese physician also interrogated the patient and his family and—interestingly enough—interpreted the patient's dreams in relation to his illness.

A study of therapy as advocated in the *Classic* indicates the ever-present preoccupation with the laws of the universe:

In order to effect a cure and relief, one must not err towards the laws of Heaven, nor towards those of the Earth, for they form a unit.

Accordingly, the physician was told that the 5 elements were paralleled by 5 methods of treatment. Since, however, disease was not a natural phenomenon—the earliest and wisest inhabitants of the earth were reputed to have been entirely free from it because of their virtuous mode of life—these 5 methods were not developed simultaneously; they evolved successively with the increasing lawlessness of succeeding generations.

The *Classic* reports that the 1st method of treatment evolved by the Chinese was the cure of the spirit. This method, strangely reminiscent of the most modern medical theories, consisted in helping the patient find the right way of life, that is, in finding contentment, repose and in avoiding excesses and ambition: "Those who are satisfied with their station in life will rise above it."

The 2nd method of treatment was the nourishment of the body. To do this correctly, the physician had to consult the 5 elements and the various factors related to them. The *Classic* states that "each of the diseases of the four seasons and the five main organs reacts to that one of the five flavours to which (each of the seasons and the organs) responds." The 5 flavours—sour, bitter, sweet, pungent and salty—were held to be related in this order to the liver, the heart, the spleen, the lungs and the kidneys, and were supposed to have in this connection a binding, strengthening, retarding, dispersing and softening effect upon the intestines. This rather rigid scheme of concordances of the 5 flavours was softened by the statement that in general the produce of each season and each particular region constituted the ideal nourishment.

The next method of treatment advocated by the *Classic* concerns the true effects of medicines. Here again we are referred to the 5 predominant qualities contained in each of them; but the subject is treated too generally to repay detailed study. Beyond the mention of the existence of medicines, which were derived from the animal, vegetable and mineral kingdoms and held to represent a mixture of Heaven and Earth, we do not find an elaboration of the matter.

The Yellow Emperor's Classic, like most other later works dealing with internal medicine, does not contain much pharmacological information, which is reserved for the numerous treatises specifically devoted to the description of China's famous materia medica. The earliest of these *Pen Tsao* or "Herbal" was attributed to the authorship of Shen Nung, the "Divine Husbandman," another of China's legendary emperors.

The 4th method instructs the physician on how to combat disorder of the bowels and the viscera; this was done mainly by massage and by insistence upon proper evacuation of the bowels and elimination of the waters.

The methods of treatment so far discussed presuppose an

attitude of watchful waiting on the part of the physician. The guidance towards proper conduct, the establishment of a correct diet, the designation of a few medicines and the insistence upon daily evacuation appear to us as an encouragement of the healing power of nature rather than as an active means of curing disease. It is the 5th method of treatment, however, that enables the physician to take an active part in combating illness; and, since this method represents the most important expression of universalistic philosophy as applied to actual medical practice, I should like here to devote some time to its description. This method is the application of acupuncture and moxibustion.

Acupuncture, also known as "needling," consists in the insertion of needles of various shapes, sizes and materials into specific points of the body, the extremities and even the head. These needles may be withdrawn immediately, left in situ for some time, or rotated a number of times, depending on the nature of the ailment. Moxibustion, or moxa treatment, is practiced by applying to the skin combustible cones of the dried and powdered leaves of artemisia vulgaris; these cones are then ignited and allowed to burn down to the skin until a small blister forms. Both remedies are of great antiquity and must have been well known as early as the time of the composition of *The Yellow Emperor's Classic,* for the book deals with refinements of procedure, rather than with basic instructions concerning their use. The cosmological significance of both these methods of treatment lies in the location and number of acupuncture and moxibustion spots, and in the motivation given to their use.

In order to understand the theories behind acupuncture and moxibustion we must bring to mind again the basic concepts of pathology and physiology as discussed above. Disease was believed to arise out of an imbalance of the dual force Yin and Yang, leading to an obstruction or insufficiency of either element within the 12 main vessels which were held to be connected with the various parts of organs of the body. Significantly, there are 365 points where these vessels rise to the surface of the body and thus present the spots for acupuncture and moxibustion. The effect of the insertion of the needles and the blistering of the moxa cone is to create openings for the relief of congestion caused by a plethora of Yin and Yang. According to the *Classic,* acupuncture and moxibustion were applied for a vast variety of complaints, and especially for acute pains produced by rheumatism and neuralgic conditions, cramps and colics; both were recommended in cases of mental disturbance:

> Ch'i Po said: "In order to puncture one must enter the meridian repeatedly, and one uses the moment in inhalation to push the needle. Hence, in order to nourish and care for the spirit and mind one must be aware of the appearances of the body: whether it is fat or thin, whether the blood, the vital essences, the constitution and the breath are flourishing or deteriorating."

> The Emperor said: "How wonderful this reasoning! To bring into agreement man's body with Yin and Yang, the two principles in nature, and with the four seasons; his echoing of want and fullness, his response to the most subtle influences. . . ."

The description of these various methods of therapy concludes the discussion of the fundamentals of Chinese medicine. But these fundamentals, conceived in the dawn of China's existence and recorded centuries before our era, have not been relegated to the realm of history. In spite of the advent of Western practices, the Chinese have never completely ceased to employ their own art of healing, mainly because it continued to fit into their specific philosophy of life, but also because it appears that in frequent cases it was good medicine. Even though many Chinese doctors and patients of more recent centuries may no longer have been consciously aware of the cosmological basis of their treatments, works like *The Yellow Emperor's Classic* and the many that followed provided such detailed methods of procedure that individual reasoning was unnecessary.

The thought of man's origin and composition as part of the universe never, however, quite left the Chinese mind and was the only existing theory until the introduction by Western scientists of the study of anatomy and the practice of surgery. Even in Japan, where Chinese medicine was adopted in the 6th century A.D., and retained until well into the 10th century, there can be found a deep-rooted and unquestioning belief in the analogy between man and the universe. This is true even for a man like Kagawa Genetsu, the author of the first enlightened text-book on midwifery, who is generally spoken of as the founder of Japanese obstetrics. His work was based on personal study and observation, but obviously there had never arisen an occasion for him to dissect an embryo. Thus, in the *San Ron* (1765) he described the nature and composition of an embryo aborted during the first 3 months. Such an embryo, he stated, was round; if it was cut apart it would show the 5 colours representing the 5 elements. This, Kagawa held, furnished absolute proof that man was composed of water, fire, air, earth and wood, the 5 elements composing the universe.

If the ancient theoretical foundations were kept alive, it is even less surprising that the methods of treatment have continued to be practiced in China and Japan. The examination of the pulse has remained the main diagnostic method of the typical Chinese and Japanese practitioner. And, while the materia medica has become richer and more varied than had been described in *The Yellow Emperor's Classic,* it is still applied according to the same principles. Acupuncture and moxibustion, too, have remained in uninterrupted use. A Chinese treatise, the Ming T'ang Ching (probably composed during the Sung dynasty, 960-1279 A.D.), translated into Japanese as the *Mei-do-kiyo,* elaborated on the instructions given in *The Yellow Emperor's Classic.* The most graphic description of these practices from a Western point of view is contained in *The History of Japan* . . . 1690-92 by Engelbert Kaempfer, a German physician who was attached to the Dutch settlement in Deshima in the late 17th century.

At present the preoccupation with ancient Chinese medical methods no longer seems to be the exclusive domain of the indigenous practitioner. Articles, books and numerous personal communications bring to light the fact that Western and Western-trained physicians have begun a scientific investigation into the actual value of these methods which have remained in practice for more than 2500 years.

If the history of *The Yellow Emperor's Classic* is compared with that of the *Corpus Hippocraticum,* which originated at about the same time, a curious and somewhat contradictory development may be noted. The works of the Greek tradition were composed to serve as text-books for the practitioner, yet the practical value of their contents was superseded centuries ago. Apart from their significance for the medical historian, the value of these works has for centuries consisted in creating for the Western physician the moral and ethical concept of the ideal physician. On the other hand, from the preceding discussion it should be evident that China's earliest book concerned with the art of healing was never meant to be a mere text-book of medicine, but rather a treatise on the philosophy of nature; and yet it was taken over by the physician, not as a guide towards an ideal of life, but as a help for the actual practice of medicine. It is not within the scope of this paper to make further comparison between the literary monuments of two such divergent traditions, but it is hoped that the modern doctor, whose spiritual ancestor is Hippocrates, and who today is trained in clinical research and the psychosomatic aspect of disease, will not fail to discover the philosophical wisdom of *The Yellow Emperor's Classic of Internal Medicine.*

REFERENCES

Diamond, E. G.: "Ward rounds with an acupuncturist," *New England Journal of Medicine* 272 (1965), 575-577.

Hume, Edward: *The Chinese Way of Medicine,* Baltimore, Johns Hopkins Univ. Press, 1940.

Palos, Stephan: *The Chinese Art of Healing,* New York, Herder and Herder, 1971.

Rall, Jutta: *Die vier grossen Medizinschulen der Mongolenzeit,* Stand und Entwicklung der chinesischen Medizin in der Chin — und — Yüan — Zeit. Münchener Ostasiatische Studien, Band 4. Wiesbaden, Franz Steiner Verlag, 1970.

Veith, I.: "Acupuncture therapy, past and present: verity or delusion," *JAMA* 180 (1962), 478-484.

Veith, I.: "The beginnings of modern Japanese obstetrics," *Bulletin of the History of Medicine* 25 (1951), 45-59.

Veith, Ilza: *Some Philosophical Concepts of Early Chinese Medicine,* Transaction No. 4. *The Indian Institute of Culture,* Basavanjudi, Bangalore, India, 1950.

Veith, Ilza: *The Yellow Emperor's Classic of Internal Medicine,* transl. with an introd. study. Berkeley, Univ. of California Press, 1966.

Chapter 2

TRADITIONAL MEDICINE IN MODERN CHINA: SOCIAL, POLITICAL, AND CULTURAL ASPECTS

Ralph C. Croizier

T HIS PAPER, TOO, will be part of the "historical background" for this symposium, but my historical vistas are limited to the last few decades instead of the thousands of years Dr. Veith has covered. However, by "modern China" I do not just mean the Chinese People's Republic, but rather China since the middle or late 19th century by which time the age-old Chinese civilization, of which traditional medicine was an integral part, had started to disintegrate under the impact of Western pressure.

One convenient way of finding a starting date might be to look for the appearance of the term "Chinese medicine" in China. Although the traditional medicine was several thousand years old, it only acquired the name "Chinese medicine" after the Chinese became aware of the very different medical system brought by the West. That they naturally called "Western medicine," while their own traditional medical system then began to be called "Chinese medicine."

This bit of historical semantics is important for what I am attempting in this paper—to put "Chinese medicine" into the larger context of the sweeping political, social, and cultural revolution that has transformed China and to show how some of the pressures generated in that revolution have influenced the nature of traditional medicine in modern China.

30

The first aspect of this larger context that must be noted is the strong ambivalence modern Chinese nationalism has shown towards the nation's traditional culture. On the one hand, the birth of political nationalism has required a rejection of the age-old essentially cultural definition of "China." Moreover, the ruthless logic of modernization has forced abandonment, willing or unwilling, of many of the distinctive forms, values, and institutions which comprised Confucian China. But, on the other hand, modern nationalism has also fostered a more intense, particularistic attachment to specifically Chinese cultural traditions. With China's cultural identity threatened by the massive flood of Western cultural importations, modern Chinese have been torn between the need to reject the traditional culture as outmoded and the desire to prize it as Chinese.

Medicine has been one of the more striking examples of this tension. Here we find intersecting two of the main compulsions in modern Chinese nationalism — the drive for national power through mastery of modern science, and the effort to reaffirm the autonomy and creativity of Chinese culture. There is a consistency to both of these drives running throughout all of modern Chinese history from the nineteenth century Confucian self-strengtheners, who sought to save the old world which was their very being, to Communist social revolutionaries who seek to remake man and society in a new image. The drive for modern science and its fruits (from steamships to nuclear weapons) is the more obvious, but the overwhelming triumph of scientism in twentieth century China has not weakened the Chinese desire to own the cultural ground they stand on. This is evident in the many tortuous rationalizations attempting to show that the adoption of Western institutions, values, and ideologies has not meant cultural surrender to the invading West—that modern Chinese still make their own history according to a Chinese formula and not merely following a Western cultural blueprint.

It has been this latter compulsion that has made so unlikely a field as medicine an arena for cultural and intellectual controversy. The beginning of this controversy can be traced back to the early years of this century when the gradual introduction of Western medicine threatened to eclipse and supplant the native tradition in medicine. While the old medical practices persisted among the vast majority of the population, the new Republic's decision to sponsor only modern medicine was an augury of things to come. More menacing than any proclamations of the weak and ineffective national government, however, was the bitter hostility manifested toward the old medicine by the new generation of radical young intellectuals.

For this generation, usually identified with the May Fourth Movement of 1919, traditional medicine stood out as a particularly noxious symbol of the traditional culture—backwards, superstitious, irrational—which had to be destroyed for China to survive in the modern world. To men who saw "science" as a panacea for China's manifold ills it was intolerable that this hoary, unscientific tradition should be allowed to survive in an area so central to science, human welfare, and national strength as medicine. With a violent rhetoric common to his times one of the nationalistic new youth, Chang Tsung-liang, summed up the charges against Chinese medicine:

> The hollow-breasted and humpbacked, the pale-faced and slender-limbed, consequently the devastating epidemic, the high death rate, the lack of strong character and national morale, the pessimistic belief in destiny . . . the award of the very title of 'The Far Eastern Sick Person' — these are the direct gifts of the old style medicine to China.

Paradoxically it was at this juncture—with cultural iconoclasm at full tide and science riding its crest—that there arose the first serious efforts to preserve the traditional medical system in a modern context. To be sure, there had been some tentative gropings in that direction in the early years of the century. Most notable, were the efforts of Ting Fu-pao, a traditional scholar with some modern medical education, who tried to harmonize the two medical systems in a series of books he published in Shanghai. On the level of institutional change, the traditionally highly diffuse native medical profession had responded to the government's patronage of Western medicine by forming a "Committee for Saving Chinese Medicine" when threatened by a government decision to make Western medicine the basis of the approved medical curriculum. However, the real impetus behind a much more determined effort to "save Chinese medicine" did not come from traditional scholars or the old-style practitioners themselves. It came rather from twentieth century intellectuals and politicians whose motives were essentially as modern as those of the radical iconoclasts who so ruthlessly damned the indigenous medical system.

These conflicting attitudes towards tradition, and towards traditional medicine in particular, were a part of that great sea of change in Chinese intellectual perspectives whereby China as a cultural entity—the only true form of civilization—disappeared in favor of China as a nation among other competing, and threatening, nation-states. As a culture China had been impervious to political threat—conquest dynasties might come and go so long as they did not disturb the cultural basis of Chinese civilization. As a nation, now that pretentions to absolute cultural superiority had been shattered, China could freely part with her traditional culture if it impeded the rapid modernization which survival demanded. Freely, and yet not so freely. For, while the logic of the new nationalism freed modern Chinese from unswerving loyalty to the old culture, nationalistic emotions engendered new loyalties to what was distinctively Chinese. Thus, modern nationalism by the nineteen twenties offered license both to cultural iconoclasm and to cultural nationalism—the one to destroy the old culture as harmful to the nation, the other to cherish it as the unique product and hallmark of the national genius.

In medicine this meant that, while critics like Chang Tsung-liang were rejecting traditional Chinese medicine in toto, a new generation of conservatives sought ways to save it from extinction. They differed basically from pure traditionalists in that these new conservatives had a healthy respect for Western science and much of Western medicine. They also frankly recognized many of the shortcomings of the native medical system and stressed the need to adopt the organizational and institutional forms of modern medicine. But unlike the cultural radicals, they did not want Chinese medicine, as a system of medical thought and practice, to disappear before the inexorable advance of scientific Western medicine. They insisted that Chinese medicine possessed a core of precious and unique value which, purged of excrescences and supplemented with science, must be preserved. Moreover, the preservation of this "national essence" in medicine would offer reassurance to a shaken national confidence that in at least this one area of science China could produce something of value on her own.

The first important political patron of "reformed" or "scientificized" Chinese medicine was the warlord governor of Shansi province, Yen Hsi-shan. In 1921 he set up a "Research Society for the Reform of Chinese Medicine" with the ambitious purpose of combining the best features of Chinese and Western medicine in order to produce a new system of medicine both scientific and still distinctively Chinese. Yen was not very clear about exactly how this would be done, and the "research" of his society did little to clarify the problem. But the appeal of this vague syncretic formula (as with so many other suggested syncretisms between East and West) was considerable to those Chinese who wanted China to become modern but were dubious about abandoning so much of Chinese culture in the process.

Accordingly, in the next decade there emerged a number of similar organizations in various parts of China. More modern-minded traditional doctors naturally played a large role in these, although non-medical intellectual and political luminaries, such as the veteran Nationalist revolutionary Chang Ping-ling, were also intimately involved in their efforts. It was not until after the establishment of the Nationalist Government in 1927, however, that all this grew into a serious national movement.

The specific impetus to form a nation-wide organization of defenders of Chinese medicine was provided by a resolution adopted by the new Nanking Government's Ministry of Health calling for the step-by-step elimination of all old-style medical practice in China. This provoked a great outcry not only among traditional practitioners, who saw their livelihood threatened, but also among cultural conservatives in general, who saw this as yet another instance of the national culture being swept away by the craze for things modern and foreign. Such sentiments were sufficiently widespread in the higher levels of the ruling Nationalist Party itself to have the resolution quickly shelved. More important, out of the uproar came a new nation-wide organization, The Institute for National Medicine (Kuo-i Kuan), founded to defend China's own "national" medicine against further threats.

Probably the most articulate (certainly the most politically influential) spokesman for this organization and for the reformed Chinese medicine viewpoint in general, was the important Nationalist politician and ideologue, Ch'en Kuo-fu. As part of the general turn towards a politically and culturally more conservative outlook within the Nationalist Party after 1927, Ch'en had risen rapidly to great power in Party affairs under the aegis of Chiang Kai-shek. A militant nationalist and firmly dedicated to making China a strong power, he naturally emphasized China's need for modern science and technology, including scientific medicine. But, like many other conservative nationalists, he balked at the liberals' and radicals' insistence that this required complete social and cultural revolution. Such thorough-going "Westernization" was an affront to national pride, and we find Ch'en Kuo-fu denouncing as unpatriotic those modernizers who "superstitiously venerate" everything foreign and lack faith in anything of China's own cultural tradition. He offered medicine as one example of this despicable attitude—despicable because it weakened Chinese national self-confidence. And, also, a particularly important example, for here the Chinese tradition had something to offer in that field where modern China's cultural indebtedness to the West was heaviest—science.

Ch'en did not attempt to portray traditional medicine in China as purely scientific. Obviously it was not, and obviously it needed considerable reform to become so. But he did insist that in its fundamentals the indigenous medical system was compatible with science (for it was based on empirically determined experience, the very essence of science) and that it possessed a unique body of medical wisdom that could not be allowed to perish.

On the level of practical techniques and materia medica a convincing case could readily be made; on its claims to respect as an integral "system" of medicine, the task was much more difficult. Ch'en tried valiantly to explain, or explain away, the traditional medical theories of *Yin-Yang* and the five elements as no more than symbolic terminology for natural physiological processes, but without notable success. Similarly, he and other apologists for Chinese medicine were baffled by how to explain the important therapeutical technique of acupuncture in terms acceptable to a modern, scientific audience. The central dilemma lay in reconciling the fundamentally different principles and methodology of modern science with these ancient medical concepts, a dilemma which has remained the most formidable obstacle to the proposed synthesis of Chinese and Western medicine. To cut away too much of the native medical theory would destroy its integrity as a "Chinese" system of medicine; to retain it made the expropriation of "science" (and all the values associated with it) extremely difficult. As Ch'en's critics pointed out, if you replace the old medical ideas with universal scientific principles, why call it "Chinese" medicine?

But logic need not overrule emotional needs, so Ch'en and others like him continued to strive for a reformed Chinese medicine which would satisfy their attachments both to science and to a Chinese identity. Ch'en was particularly insistent on the institutional reform of traditional medicine to reach this goal. Professional medical associations, research centers, hospitals, medical schools—all the organizational features of modern medicine—were urgently required to correct the sorry state of actual medical practice in China. Implied in this was the common conservative assumption that behind a framework of foreign-inspired institutional change a viable Chinese essence could be preserved. The value of this essence, once it had been properly "put in order," need not be confined to China. In their more euphoric moments Ch'en and his colleagues waxed enthusiastic on what a blessing the new Chinese medicine, combining the best of East and West, would be to all mankind. What better proof could be offered to a doubting world of China's continued cultural creativity? More to the point, what better method could be found to ease the modern Chinese sense of cultural indebtedness? "Scientificized" Chinese medicine would pay back the West in its own scientific coin.

Throughout the nineteen-thirties and forties the Institute for National Medicine and its adherents continued to clamor for active government sponsorship of their program. They were consistently opposed by liberal intellectuals outside of the government and by the modern-medicine oriented Ministry of Health within it. The result was pretty much of a standoff. The Institute for National Medicine was unable on its own to go very far in providing the medical schools, research centers, and hospitals its program envisioned—or in getting the government to underwrite them. On the other hand, it was able to block any attempts by the Ministry of Health to regulate or restrict the practice of traditional medicine. Thus, throughout the National Government period the two medical worlds—old and new, Chinese and Western—remained sharply divided and mutually hostile, despite the efforts of persons like Ch'en Kuo-fu to synthesize the two in a new, and superior, Chinese medicine.

Up to 1949 there was a certain logic or consistency to the alignment of opinion over the Chinese medicine question. The proponents of indigenous medicine were generally on the conservative side of political and cultural questions; their opponents could usually be classified as "progressives" or "liberals." Under the People's Republic, however, there has been a curious reversal of roles with a ruthlessly modern and scientific Communist regime taking up the cause of preserving a Chinese medical identity and condemning skeptics for unprogressive and unpatriotic thought. Again, we must turn to the general history of modern China and of Chinese Communism for an explanation.

The first generation of Chinese Marxists in the early nineteen twenties fully shared the cultural iconoclasm prevalent among the young intellectuals of their time. But in the ensuing decades, after the Communist movement had been driven from the urban centers of Western cultural influence and faced with the problem of how to survive in a rural setting, the Party gradually adopted a less hostile policy towards the native medicine and its practitioners. Originally, this was clearly no more than making virtue out of necessity—using traditional medicine to alleviate the critical shortage of modern doctors and medical facilities. Despite misgivings by some of the Communist Party's medical cadres, this was apparently in line with the strong emphasis in Maoist strategy on adapting and using native resources for modern ends. As Mao himself explained at a wartime conference in Yenan, the old-style doctors were not scientific but they could be trained and used for the people's health. The Communists' medical leadership was enjoined to use, and improve, this indigenous medical resource.

Accession to national power in 1949 took the Communists out of the hills of Yenan into the major urban centers, but it did not solve their basic medical problem. China had some first-class modern medical establishments (notably the Rockefeller-financed Peking Union Medical College) and a core of highly trained medical leaders, but in quantitative terms the situation was still critical. There were perhaps 15,000 modern-trained doctors for a population of over 500 million. It required no great extension of Maoist pragmatism to continue the policy already in effect before 1949, even though some modern doctors might grumble about concessions to quackery and superstition.

For the first four or five years of the People's Republic the main thrust of policy towards Chinese medicine was in organizing and controlling its numerous practitioners (probably upwards of half a million throughout the country) and giving them some of the rudiments of modern medicine and public health. The first goal was achieved through "Health-worker Unions" and cooperative-type "United Clinics," the second by organizing short-term "Improvement Classes." Despite a certain amount of favorable propaganda about the usefulness of the old-style doctors and the masses' trust in them, there was little indication in this period that traditional medicine was intended for anything other than essentially a stopgap purpose until sufficient numbers of scientifically trained doctors were available.

By 1954, however, a new theme began to impinge upon the

early emphasis to learn everything from Soviet medical experience. This was an increased respect for the "medical legacy
of the motherland" and warnings to modern-medicine trained
public health authorities that this legacy must not be neglected
in developing the new "people's medicine." Abstract warnings
were then replaced by specific charges against specific persons
highly placed in the Ministry of Health. The two best known
targets for a systematic campaign of public denunciation were
Ho Ch'eng, the Deputy Minister of Health, and Wang Pin,
Minister of Health in Manchuria. The ideological crimes they
were charged with consisted of despising and belittling Chinese
medicine in favor of total reliance on Western methods. In
practice, this allegedly had caused them to interpret Party
directives on combining Chinese and Western medicine merely
to mean that old-style doctors should learn some modern medicine. They would then serve as auxiliaries to the Western style
doctors until enough of the latter were trained to take over all
medical practice. Wang Pin was particularly denounced for re-
ferring to the native tradition as "feudal medicine," and great
pains were now taken to show how medicine was "relatively free
from class-nature" or, in any event, was the product of the ac-
cumulated wisdom of the Chinese masses and hence, by definition, good.

Apart from a sudden upsurge of nationalistic sentiment about
China's own glorious medical achievements, the most serious
aspect of the Party's new interest in Chinese medicine was the
linking of medical attitudes to ideological correctness. The
suspicion of pro-Western bourgeois influences in the modern
medical profession was perfectly natural, for the overwhelming
majority of its leadership had been educated either in Europe,
America, or missionary founded institutions in China. During the
first few years after 1949 a heavy dose of Soviet medicine had
been seen as the best antidote to these unfortunate connections
and their ideological influence. But the question of "bourgeois
tendencies" (i.e. separation from the masses and independence
from Party control) was found to be more complex than simply
pre-1949 capitalist connections. Rather, it was an integral part of

the larger dilemma of how to treat the technical elite—the dilemma usually posed in terms of "red vs. expert." These experts (doctors included) were vitally important to the Party's goals of modernization and industrialization, but giving them the high social status which education traditionally had conferred in China, plus the *de facto* power which their importance to modernization demanded, went strongly against the egalitarian social goals of the revolution and against the Party cadres' ("the reds") untrammeled exercise of their new power. The mid-nineteen-fifties saw intensified efforts to curb the emergence of a new privileged technocratic class culminating in the triumph of the "mass line" during the Great Leap Forward.

The emphasis on modern doctors studying traditional medicine, starting in 1954, should be seen as part of these efforts to control the technical intelligentsia. Neither Ho Ch'eng nor Wang Pin could be convincingly accused of direct contamination by Western capitalist influences; both were long-time Party members with Soviet medical education. But they did represent (even within the Party) the tendency of "the experts" to free themselves from direct political control. This was their chief crime, and this was why a correct attitude towards Chinese medicine became the touchstone for a modern doctor's acceptance of Communist Party leadership in medical affairs.

Of course, the reappraisal of Chinese medicine also had important consequences for the actual development of medicine in China. There was a very considerable increase in the Government's expenditures on hospitals, clinics, and schools for Chinese medicine. More significant for the now clearly enunciated policy of fostering a true synthesis of the two medical systems, Chinese-style doctors and wards for Chinese medicine were incorporated into most of the major hospitals of China. Actually this created more of a parallel system of medical treatment in China's medical institutions than the desired "combined therapy." Complaints from both types of doctors and repeated exhortations from official spokesmen indicated that such integration was easier to decree than to achieve. Nevertheless, as foreign visitors frequently remarked, venerable herbalists and acupuncture specialists did become regular fixtures in the most modern medical facilities.

Foreign observers have been even more startled by the changes in medical education. By the mid-nineteen-fifties Chinese medicine had become a required subject in all modern medicine schools, and practicing Western-style physicians were pressured to enroll in spare time courses in Chinese medicine. Finally, up to 2,000 doctors at a time were withdrawn from regular practice for three years of full-time study of traditional medicine. Remembering the still critical shortage of modern-trained physicians, this substantial diversion of scarce human resources to Chinese medicine is the most solid evidence of the seriousness with which the Communist government took its policy uniting the two medicines.

The emphasis on Chinese medicine and criticism of Western-style doctors reached its peak with the great upsurge of ideological fervor in the Great Leap Forward of late 1958. The indigenous medical system, and especially its popular folkloristic features, lent itself very well to the depreciation of technical expertise at this time. After all, if an engineer could learn from a coolie, and an agronomist from an old peasant, why not have a modern medical specialist learn from a native herbalist? With the "mass line" in ascendancy, science was no esoteric monopoly of the highly educated few. Enormous numbers of home prescriptions were collected to prove the wealth of medical wisdom resident in the Chinese people, and dubious modern doctors were exhorted to use traditional remedies in their own practice. As the common slogan ran, "Western-style doctors should learn from Chinese-style doctors"—a direct reversal of their roles before 1954.

But as the heaven-storming spirit of the Great Leap waned amid economic setbacks and political difficulties the high tide of enthusiasm for Chinese medicine also subsided. By the early 1960's the increased attention to technical expertise for economic recovery was reflected in medicine by more emphasis on sophisticated modern medicine, less on the more popular aspects of traditional medicine. For example, the articles on acupuncture, herbal remedies, and the relation of both to the thought of Mao Tse-tung which had briefly flooded the prestigious *Chinese Medical Journal* in 1958-59 disappeared in the next few years. All that remained were relatively modest claims, by modern surgeons, of success in using Chinese-style mobile splints for setting fractures. Similarly in the popular press surgery, especially the rejoining of severed limbs, became the best publicized accomplishment of the Chinese medical world.

This did not mean any formal change of official policy. Integration or synthesis of the two medical systems remained the announced goal and institutional support for Chinese medicine in hospitals, research centers, and schools. But there is considerable indirect contemporary evidence, confirmed by the charges subsequently levelled in the Cultural Revolution, that during the first half of the 1960's Chinese medicine was not so much being integrated with Western medicine as it was being relegated to a supplementary and somewhat inferior position. For one thing, despite the support of research centers and training of dual system doctors, there were no announcements of research breakthroughs on the theoretical level in explaining the principles behind traditional therapeutics in scientific terms. In medical education the schools for training new Chinese-style doctors were only a fraction of those giving Western medical training. And in medical practice, although Chinese medicine evidently remained very popular, especially in the countryside, it was generally practiced alongside of, not integrated with, Western medicine.

All of this suggests a tendency for integrated Chinese medicine to suffer from the same problem that integrated Ayurveda has encountered in India—erosion of its theoretical basis in an attempt to rationalize and systematize it for standardized teaching and *de facto* relegation to second-class or paramedical status by scientifically trained public health authorities. In other words, the powerful solvent of modern science threatened to dissolve the theoretical basis of Chinese medicine and leave an assortment of remedies and procedures that might be of considerable adaptive value in providing public health care but would hardly constitute an integral medical system.

In Communist China once again it was an external, political development that checked this tendency. We refer to the Great

Proletarian Cultural Revolution. The first sign of what that cataclysmic upheaval would mean for the medical world came in 1965 when Mao Tse-tung himself expressed serious dissatisfaction with the way medical policy was developing and under the slogan "doctors to the countryside" called for a major reordering of priorities. Of course, village-level medical care has been a basic public health problem all along, but it very soon became apparent that it was also a political question. As it would emerge in the rhetoric of the Cultural Revolution, it was part of the struggle between "the two lines"—the counterrevolutionary reactionary line of Liu Shao-chi and his henchmen in favoring expensive specialized facilities for an urban elite versus the socialist mass line of Mao Tse-tung in advocating basic medical care for the broad peasant masses. Or, in somewhat deflated terms, the issue was high-level education and specialized medical research for a relative few versus spreading China's medical resources as broadly as possible across the vast countryside.

According to subsequent Red Guard allegations the medical authorities initially attempted to resist the scattering of highly trained personnel from major medical centers into remote villages. But with the full-scale eruption of the Cultural Revolution in the summer of 1966 all resistance was impossible. China's medical establishment came under the same attack for being alienated from the masses as did the rest of the Party and Government apparatus. Instead of research institutions, medical colleges, and highly-skilled specialists, the medical showpiece of the Cultural Revolution was the village based "bare-foot doctor."

A brief examination of who and what the bare-foot doctors are will reveal the role Chinese medicine has played in all of this. As the picturesque name applied to them suggests, the bare-foot doctors are not highly trained physicians using the latest in scientific medical equipment. They are practitioners with little or no formal medical education recruited on the local level for part-time medical work in their own native villages. As such, they must rely heavily on local resources, both material and intellectual. In medicine this means heavy reliance on the indigenous Chinese medical tradition. Though the bare-foot doctors are not purely practitioners of traditional Chinese medicine, and most apparently have only minimal training in its theoretical principles, in practice they commonly use acupuncture and herbal remedies. This fits perfectly into the Cultural Revolution's general stress on local self-reliance and depreciation of bureaucratic structures and formal expertise.

Chinese medicine has also proved well adapted to the ideological goals of the Cultural Revolution. Innumerable cure stories, some verging on the miraculous, have appeared testifying to the efficacy of Chinese medicine when administered along with a large dose of the "Thought of Chairman Mao." The typical case is of a poor peasant or worker whose malady was dismissed as incurable by "famous bourgeois specialists" before he was treated by a People's Liberation Army medical corpsman or barefoot doctor. This "people's doctor," inspired by the Thought of Chairman Mao and determined to serve the people at all costs, customarily cures the patient through heroic acupuncture. Heroic because the doctor dares to innovate by using new techniques, such as deeper insertion of needles, and also because he first experiments on himself disregarding the pain. The cured patient inevitably profusely expresses his gratitude to Chairman Mao.

Similarly in institutional terms, Chinese medicine has been central to the major development to come out of the Cultural Revolution. In late 1968 the national press began to feature reports on the recently established rural "Cooperative Medical System." Based on either the commune or production brigade, it is a local cooperative health service bringing socialized medicine to the countryside for the first time. Members pay an annual subscription and then only nominal fees for treatment. Again, local self-reliance with minimal dependence upon county or urban hospitals is the keynote, and again this means a great deal of reliance on indigenous Chinese medicine.

It is too early, and information is too fragmentary, to assess the significance of this new institution for building a socialized rural health care system from the bottom up rather than from the top down. There certainly are questions about the quality of medical care in modern or traditional medicine. It seems unlikely that rural clinics and bare-foot doctors can replace modern hospitals and medical college graduates. But they may complement the latter and in terms of treating common minor ailments, spreading basic public hygiene, and even teaching birth control in the villages may provide important services that otherwise would not be available for years if not decades.

As for the reorganized urban medical colleges and humbler rural medical schools that are emerging out of the Cultural Revolution, their revolutionized new curricula stress integrating the study of Chinese and Western medicine. Thus both at the village level and in major medical centers Chinese medicine currently is very prominent.

Only time will tell whether the cooling of the ideological fervor of the Cultural Revolution will cause a cooling of the enthusiasm for Chinese medicine along the pattern of what happened after the Great Leap Forward. For the present it is important to note that the popularized Chinese medicine in vogue today differs considerably from traditional Chinese medicine—and not just because its practitioners carry the little red book instead of *The Yellow Emperor's Classic.*

This is because, despite all the praise for the wonder-working ability of acupuncture or herbal remedies, the new practitioners of Chinese medicine are not being trained in its underlying theoretical basis. All the emphasis is on practice and treating common disease. The basic sciences in modern medical education have been reduced, but so has the background training in Chinese medicine. An article on "new acupuncture theory," for instance, dismisses the need to learn all 365 needling points since only several dozen are commonly used. It makes no reference to the *ching-lo* anatomical system that provides the rationale for acupuncture. Divorced from its theoretical basis, it becomes an assortment of empirically applied remedies, not a medical system.

Therefore I feel, as I did in 1966, that the future of Chinese medicine as an integral system is highly problematic. The tumultuous events of the last four years have given selected popular aspects of traditional medicine great prominence in the contemporary Chinese medical scene, but they have also pushed it towards a popularization and integration with Western medicine which all the more undermines its autonomy as a medical system. In a sense synthesis is taking place, but it is all at the level of practice. It is not the kind of theoretical synthesis that earlier nationalistic advocates of "scientificized Chinese medicine" wanted and that the Communists themselves championed in the 1950s.

This does not mean that specific practices from the old medical system will soon disappear. Nor does it imply that they cannot have great adaptive value in meeting very real health problems. I think it does suggest that the nationalistic ideology of many of our medical revivalists—the dream of a new medical system that was uniquely Chinese in its theoretical foundations as well as its practical application—is not likely to be realized.

But the name "Chinese medicine" will probably be with us for some time. And so long as it is, so long as there is a concern that medicine in China not be all "Western medicine," the kind of non-medical factors discussed in this paper are going to be relevant to the future of Chinese medicine—and to the future of medicine in China.

REFERENCES

Croizier, R. C.: "Traditional medicine in Communist China: Science, Communism and Cultural Nationalism," *China Quarterly* 23 (1965), 1-27.

Gould, Sidney H., ed.: *Sciences in Communist China*, Washington, D.C., A.A.A.S., 1961.

Kwok, D. W. Y.: *Scientism in Chinese Thought, 1900-1950*, New Haven, Yale Univ. Press, 1965.

Levenson, Joseph R.: *Confucian China and its Modern Fate: the Problem of Intellectual Continuity*, Berkeley, Univ. of California Press, 1958.

"Promotion of Chinese medicine in Communist China," *Union Research Service* 3 (1956), 276-298.

"Senior medical personnel and popular physicians go to the countryside," *Union Research Service* 38 (1965), 340-355.

Part III

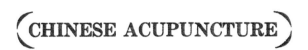

CHINESE ACUPUNCTURE

Chapter 3

THE OLD AND NEW CHINESE ACUPUNCTURE: A PREFACE

Guenter B. Risse

Traditional Chinese medicine is a great treasury and efforts should be made to develop it

—Mao Tse-tung

THE FIRST IMPETUS for our contemporary curiosity about acupuncture relates to its origin: it is a Chinese practice. As mentioned before, our previous curiosity and fascination with China and its people has suddenly resurfaced in our country. More recently, such intense desire to learn about the People's Republic has been legitimized and further fueled by the presidential visit to Peking.

A second factor in the growing interest in acupuncture can be ascribed to the current wave of anti-scientific sentiment which has engulfed a number of our contemporaries. In their perspective, Chinese acupuncture appears to be a successful method of treatment which has developed independently and seemingly transcends modern scientific medicine. The present use of acupuncture by a quarter of the world's population is used as a fact to illustrate its alleged effectiveness and serves as a vindication for other ancient and exotic practices scoffed at by modern scientific minds.

Traditionally Chinese acupuncture is a therapeutic procedure consisting in the insertion of fine needles into certain areas of the skin. The origins of this method are uncertain and can probably be linked to other attempts in primitive medicine to remove disease material or evil spirits through suction or scarifi-

49

cation. The earliest needles employed were made of flint until
the advent of metals such as bronze, silver and even gold.

Like most empirically derived procedures, the action of acupuncture had to be coherently explained in order to acquire
legitimacy and the status of a rational practice. Such an evolution
probably took place many centuries before Christ since the oldest
known Chinese text on medicine contains an elaborate explanation of the reasons for and the effects of acupuncture.

In the Yellow Emperor's Classic textbook of medicine,
probably written during the third century B.C., acupuncture
appears solidly woven into a philosophy of nature containing
Confucian and Taoist thoughts. The cosmic balance between the
two principles, the Yin and the Yang, resulted in a normal flow
of life force or Ch'i within the human body. The Ch'i was thought
to flow throughout the body along an invisible network of twelve
connecting channels or meridians, each representing a certain
month of the year. These meridians were established by linking
together specific areas of the skin selected for the insertion of
needles—the so-called acupuncture points. In the original scheme
there were 365 of these spots corresponding with the number of
days in the year.

According to the Chinese philosophical theory of disease, all
illnesses were caused by an imbalance between the Yin and the
Yang, thus affecting the flow of Ch'i. The insertion of acupuncture
needles—left in the skin for variable periods of time—was thought
to restore the lost equilibrium, possibly by allowing the escape
of the principle in excess. A variation of this procedure was to
ignite a small portion of herbs over the specified acupuncture
points instead of inserting a needle—moxibustion.

This highly schematized system of Chinese philosophical
medicine remained viable and in use for many centuries into
our own days, although the explanations of acupuncture in terms
of the Yin, Yang and Ch'i have gradually receded. Neither the
technique nor the rationale for the employment of traditional
acupuncture have undergone fundamental changes. Within the
broader context of medical history both acupuncture and moxibustion should be considered as specific instances of counter-

irritation, employed since the dawn of history, which essentially irritate, damage and even deliberately inflame certain areas of the skin in order to produce favorable systemic reactions in the body capable of throwing off disease.

Among these procedures is dry cupping, the use of a horn or cup whose air content is heated before the mouth of the vessel is applied to predetermined cutaneous regions. The partial vacuum achieved inside the cup allows a partial suction of the underlying skin with the production of spherical hematomas. In another procedure called wet cupping, small dermal incisions were made before the application of cupping vessels, allowing the discharge of serum and blood from the wound. There is an obvious similarity between Western scarification instruments and certain Chinese acupuncture needles such as the presently employed hammer or plum-blossom needle.

The deliberate production of blisters and deep burns was not exclusively done through moxibustion. The use of hot irons or needles was widespread in primitive medicine and cauterization was commonly employed for the cure of many internal illnesses down to our own time. The parallelism between medieval cautery maps and sixteenth century moxibustion and acupuncture charts is evident. Moreover, in acupuncture, heat is sometimes applied to the distal end of an inserted needle producing local blisters.

One of the physiological mechanisms underlying counter-irritation is primarily centered around reflexes linking the skin and inner organs. Every segment of the skin or dermatome is connected at the level of the spine to other nerves of the autonomic system serving specific inner organs. The various skin injuries produce local substances capable of acting as nerve transmitters. The ensuing greater local blood flow induced by these irritations is matched by a similar effect in the corresponding organs through cutaneo-visceral reflexes.

To these effects of the autonomic nervous systems can be added some hormonal changes and an increase of white blood cells associated with a stressful situation such as painful contact with a needle, blade or hot substance. Therefore, all counterirritation procedures prompt the organism into making a greater emergency response which could possibly contribute to overcoming the disease with which it is afflicted. In the absence of any pharmacologically active drugs such a reaction could make the difference between a speedier recovery from illness or the gradual deterioration of an organism whose defenses are progressively overwhelmed.

These favorable effects achieved from the various counterirritation procedures gave watchful practitioners, since time immemorial, the impression that they could be useful for their patients, and thus these methods continued to be used into our own times. Hence, I would postulate that Chinese acupuncture is another approach to healing through counter-irritation, discovered perhaps accidentally and gradually developed by trial and error as a useful form of medical treatment. In order to provide acupuncture with an acceptable rationale and thoroughly systematize the procedure, it was subsequently explained in terms of the Chinese philosophy of nature.

Although traditional acupuncture is still widely used in the rural setting of the People's Republic for treating a great variety of diseases, I honestly see no place for its use in the more affluent and technologically advanced Western nations, including our own. The relatively easy availability of many highly effective and purified drugs in our culture is to be preferred to the bodily stimulation which follows acupuncture. To transplant such an ancient and primitive healing system from its backward rural environment into our sophisticated and predominantly urban societies is either an exercise in snobbery or a reflection of total ignorance. This is not to ignore or scoff at the usefulness of traditional acupuncture in the poor villages of China. Combined with the ingestion of some pharmacologically active herbs, the method has a definite place in such a milieu considering the prevailing social, economic and cultural conditions.

The introduction of traditional Chinese acupuncture into Western Europe and Russia in the last decades only seems to confirm the dubiousness of such an import. The diseases from which the French, German and British acupuncturists claim success with their method are osteoarthritis, bronchial asthma, eczema, menstrual disorders, headaches, gastrointestinal complaints, anxiety and other conditions with a large psychosomatic component. The danger, as I see it, would be to employ Chinese acupuncture in those cases in which modern medical treatments have failed for a variety of reasons. Any subsequent improvement in these ailments then endows the procedure with an aura of panacea or "cure-all" following the erroneous logic of the post hoc, ergo propter hoc.

Since various panel members will address themselves specifically to acupuncture anesthesia, I shall only make a few remarks concerning this new and rather spectacular development. As pointed out in Prof. Crozier's paper, the Chinese authorities, after 1949, forced a merger between the ancient Chinese medical system and Western medicine. Such an imposed collaboration forced Western-trained and scientifically oriented physicians to study traditional Chinese medical practices and cooperate with the traditional healers on all levels of the health care system.

As a result of this contact, the scientifically trained physicians became aware that the placement of acupuncture needles occasionally gave rise to an apparent reflex analgesia or cessation of pain in places on the skin other than those being affected by the needles. The pain-reducing effects of acupuncture had been known for a long time, but were somewhat lost amidst all the other therapeutical claims. The analgesia obtained through acupuncture has no relationship to the cutaneo-visceral reflexes and will need a different neurophysiological explanation. The incidental discovery was quickly divorced from the traditional practices and specifically used to achieve analgesia for surgical purposes. The needles were inserted at new points, placed deeper into the skin and constantly manipulated in a rapid up and down movement with a simultaneous twirling.

Such a motion is carried out for about twenty minutes in specifically selected places of insertion before the patient acknowledges numbness in the area selected for surgery. Since each acupuncturist is only able to manipulate two needles at any one time, the same kind of stimulation can be provided by attaching a small clip to the shaft of each needle and then connecting them all to a direct-current and low voltage battery. In this manner a number of needles can be inserted and used without the disadvantages of a large number of acupuncturists crowding the operating room.

The anesthesiologists on the panel will discuss some of the obvious advantages inherent in surgery without general anesthesia. On the other hand it seems to me that consciousness has certain drawbacks which should be mentioned. For one, it means that the patient must lie absolutely still on the operating table sometimes for long hours and in uncomfortable positions. A sudden jerk or an uncontrollable cough reflex can mean disaster during the surgical procedure, especially when delicate structures such as the brain or small blood vessels are being operated upon. Moreover, it means listening to the surgeons, worrying about their progress and sharing with them moments of confusion or anxiety which can have deleterious effects on the patient's psyche.

From the preliminary reports received from eye-witnesses, we must give full credit to the stoicism and calmness exhibited by the Chinese patients who undergo major surgery with acupuncture anesthesia. There is undoubtedly a strong cultural factor responsible for the acceptance and the confidence expressed by the Chinese towards electro-acupuncture. Should the procedure be eventually adopted for anesthetic purposes in Western countries such cultural and psychological considerations will be of paramount importance. Unlike the Chinese, we in the U.S. and Europe have no millenary tradition of being pricked with needles in order to recover our health.

I would like to conclude by stressing again that the procedure now commonly called acupuncture anesthesia is a method developed and exclusively used in conjunction with modern scientific surgery as we know it. Unlike its traditional predecessor, this novel procedure is restricted to the relief of pain and the establishment of a degree of analgesia sufficient for surgical intervention without use of general anesthetics.

Therefore, there cannot and never will be an explanation of this type of acupuncture in terms of the ancient Chinese philosophy of nature. Besides, the method would hardly be of use to the traditional healers in rural China except for its implications in relieving pain, since they do not practice modern surgery. Acupuncture anesthesia will thus continue to be used in modern surgical facilities located in the various Chinese hospitals and clinics. It has the potential of becoming a scientifically acceptable procedure, quite distinct from the blanket therapeutic claims which traditional acupuncture has made in China and certain Western countries.

Our efforts in this symposium were primarily aimed at establishing a frank exchange of viewpoints between historians, anesthesiologists, surgeons and neurophysiologists. Together, representatives of these disciplines can initiate a scientific dialogue furnishing us with the necessary insight and evaluation of a novel technique for the relief of pain during and after surgery.

It is clear that the Chinese have only recently discovered the true analgesic qualities of the procedure, probably by chance, and have developed the whole method purely on empirical grounds. This is no sin if one consults the arduous and often embarrassing story of medical therapeutics. However, the time has come for a thorough scientific examination of the empirical evidence. In the meantime, let us not be carried away by the spectacular character of acupuncture anesthesia and attempt to employ it without first gaining more knowledge of its technique, effectiveness and possible complications. The safeguard and trust of our patients clearly demands this.

REFERENCES

Elliott, F. A.: "Acupuncture and other forms of counterirritation," *Trans. Stud. Coll. Phys. Phila.* 30 (1962/63), 81-84.

Peking Acupunctural Anesthesia Cooperation and Coordination Unit, "Points, meridians and the principle of acupunctural anesthesia," *Hung-ch'i* (Red Flag) No. 12, November 1, 1971 (an English translation of the article can be found in *Selections from China Mainland Magazines* 71-11, Nos. 717-18, November 29 to December 7, 1971, 79-87.)

Snow, E.: "Report from China III — Population care and control," *The New Republic* (May 1, 1971), 20-23.

Tsung-ying, L.: "Acupunctural anesthesia — its theory and practice," *Eastern Horizon* 10 (1971), 2-6.

Chapter 4

TECHNIQUES USED IN ACUPUNCTURE

James Y. P. Chen

I. Equipment

    A. Acupuncture Needles

The needles are made of gold, silver and other metals, but nowadays stainless steel needles are most commonly used. Gold and silver acupuncture needles are still quite popular in Europe, particularly in France.

In practice, three types of needles are generally employed: the *hao-chen* or needles for insertion; the seven-star or five-star dermal *pi fu chen* needles for light tapping in the area of acupuncture point or on children, and the *san ling chen* triangular needle for blood letting.

Needles for insertion *(hao-chen)* are of various lengths, 0.5, 1, 1-5, 2, 2-5, 3, 3-5, up to 6 or 7 inches, and of different thicknesses, usually of 26, 28 and 30 gauge.

The needle consists of four parts, the needle holder, the needle root (the top portion of the needle body just below the holder), the needle body and the needle tip or point.

    B. Other Essentials

Needle containers usually made of stainless steel, suitable for sterilization.

Bottles of 70 percent alcohol for sterilization of skin before needling.

Cotton balls.

II. Insertion and Withdrawal of the Needle

    A. Insertion of the Needle

As a general rule, hold the holder of the needle with the

thumb and index finger of the right hand, the middle finger being close to the end of the holder. Press the acupuncture point with the left hand and insert the needle with the right hand. Always insert the point of the needle rapidly through the skin, and then continue puncturing relatively slowly into deeper tissues.

There are generally four different types of needle insertion, depending upon the length of the needle and the location of the acupuncture point.

(1) "Pressing with the left thumbnail." — Insert the tip of the needle alongside the left thumbnail into the acupuncture point. This technique is commonly employed when short needles are used for insertion into points such as *Nei Kuan* (Pericardium 6. located between the ulna and radius of the forearm, two inches above the flexure of the wrist), *Ho Ku* (Large Intestine 4, on the dorsal surface of the hand in the angle of the first two metacarpals).

(2) "Insertion between two fingers." — Using the left thumb and index finger, squeeze a small cotton ball around the tip of the needle. As the left thumb and index finger press upon the acupuncture point, insert the needle with the right hand. This method is used most frequently when long needles are inserted into points such as *Huan Tiao* (Gall bladder 30, on the hip behind the greater trochanter).

(3) "Tauting the skin with the right hand." — Stretch the skin around the acupuncture point outward (away from the point) so as to tighten the skin to facilitate needle insertion. It is used in areas with loose skin such as the abdomen, *Tien Ch'u* (Stomach 25, at the level of the umbilicus three inches from the median line), *Kuan Yuan* (Conception Vessel 4, three inches below the umbilicus).

(4) "Compressing fold of skin with the left hand." — With the left thumb and index finger, pick up the skin surrounding the acupuncture point. Insert the needle at a slant angle. This method is usually used in areas where the skin and tissue are relatively thin such as the head; for instance, *Ing T'an* (Special point 1 on the median line in between the eyebrows).

B. Angle of Needling

The angle of the inserting needle in relation to the surface of the skin varies with the sites of the points and the objectives of treatment. Generally speaking, there are three types:

(1) 90-degree insertion. In most cases, this angle is used, that is, the needle is inserted perpendicularly to the skin surface.

(2) 45-degree insertion. This is used for most points on the chest where the tissue is thin or for those points adjacent to vital organs, such as *Lieh Chieh* (Lung 7, on the radial artery two inches above the flexure of the wrist).

(3) 15-25-degree horizontal insertion. Used on the head, face and neck where the skin and tissue are very thin, such as *Pai Hui* (Governing Vessel 20, on the median line of the head, about the vertex); *T'suan Chu* (Bladder 2, at the medial extremity of the eyebrow, one inch from the median line).

C. Withdrawal of the Needle

After proper manipulation of the inserted needle, it should be slightly twirled as it is withdrawn (do not withdraw the needle "straight out"). To avoid possible bleeding from the needling and to minimize residual pain following needle withdrawal, press against the punctured point ("hole") with a small cotton ball.

III. Choice of Points for Needling

From centuries of clinical observation, traditional Chinese medicine maintains that needling of certain points is particularly efficacious for certain ailments. The ancient Chinese have established certain general rules regarding the choice of points to be used for the treatment of various diseases. To facilitate learning, especially for the beginners, some of the basic rules have been put in rhymes or songs. The most popular one advises that for the gastro-intestinal ailments, the point of *Tsu San Li* (Stomach 36, located three inches below the patella, between the tibialis anterior and tibia) should be used; for lumbo-dorsal illnesses, *Wei Chung* (Bladder 54, located in the middle of the popliteal area upon the crease of the fold); for affections of the head and neck, *Lieh Ch'ueh* (Lung 7, on the anterior surface of the forearm on the radial artery, two inches above the flexure of the wrist); for ailments of the face and mouth, *Ho Ku* (Large intestine 4, on the dorsal surface of the hand in the angle of the first two metacarpals between the thumb and index finger); for women's or female ailments, *San Yin Chiao* (Spleen 6, located four inches above the medial malleolus, behind the tibia); for sickness of the chest cavity, *Nei Kuan* (Pericardium or Heart-Constrictor 6, located on the anterior surface of the forearm, between the ulna and radius two inches above the flexure of the wrist.

In actual practice, the acupuncturist usually combines one main point with some other sensitive spots near the source of illness. For instance, for headaches, the *Ho Ku* point on the hand is often combined with the *T'ai Yang* spot, a special point on the head, at the center of the temporal area.

IV. Tonification and Sedation

The proper application of the acupuncture technique requires needle manipulation to produce a stimulating (tonification) effect or a tranquilizing (sedation) effect at the points of insertion. Certain illnesses require a tonifying of the points while others may call for sedation.

The Chinese Law of *Pu Hsieh* governs the relations between tonification and sedation; *Pu* representing tonification and *Hsieh* representing sedation. One of the most commonly used techniques for tonification is, for example, to rotate the head of the needle by pushing the thumb forward while drawing the index finger back (clockwise) whereas in sedation the head of the needle is rotated by pushing the index finger forward while drawing the thumb back (counter-clockwise). Several other techniques such as expiration-inspiration, fast-slow, upstream-downstream can also be used to produce the tonification-sedation effect.

According to a recently published Chinese text on acupuncture used in China, the most commonly used needle manipulating techniques to produce tonifying or sedating effects are summarized in the following table:

EFFECTS PRODUCED BY THE MANIPULATION OF THE NEEDLE

	TONIFICATION (PU)	SEDATION (HSIEH)
INSERTING (CHIN-CH'EN)	INSERT SLOWLY WITH SLIGHT TWIRLING.	INSERT RAPIDLY WITH MORE TWIRLING.
TWIRLING (NIEN-CHUAN)	TWIRL THE NEEDLE BY PUSHING THE THUMB FORWARD AND WITHDRAWING THE INDEX FINGER BACK (CLOCKWISE).	TWIRL THE NEEDLE BY PUSHING THE INDEX FINGER FORWARD AND WITHDRAWING THE THUMB BACK (COUNTER-CLOCKWISE).
RAISING AND RE-INSERTING (T'I-CH'A) (BIRD-PECKING)	FIRST SHALLOW AND THEN DEEP INSERTION; REPEATEDLY USE GREATER FORCE IN INSERTING AND LIGHTER FORCE IN WITHDRAWING.	FIRST DEEP AND THEN SHALLOW INSERTION; REPEATEDLY USE GREATER FORCE IN WITHDRAWING AND LIGHTER FORCE IN INSERTING.
WITH-DRAWING (CHU-CH'EN)	WITHDRAW RAPIDLY.	WITHDRAW SLOWLY.

Direct translation from page 250 of the Chinese text, "Essentials of Chinese Acupuncture" (in Chinese) by the Editing Committee on Essentials of Acupuncture. Originally published by People's Public Health Press, Peking, 1964, and re-printed by Ta-Kwan Publishing Company, Hong Kong, 1970.

V. Basic Rules for Selection of Needling Points

The acupuncture points to be selected for treatment of a particular disease are based on the distribution and therapeutic characteristics of the points along the meridian relating to the diseased organ or part of the body. In general, there are three approaches as follows:

(1) Distant Point. — After determining the meridian and the organ affected by the ailment, certain distant points of the involved meridian on the limbs are used. For instance, *Tsu San Li* (Stomach 36) is selected for stomach aches; *Ho Ku* (Large Intestine 4) for tooth aches. This method is employed for affections of the head, face and various organs of the chest and abdomen. The so-called "distant point" technique is based on the general rule — "Points of the lower body for ailments of the upper body"

and "Points of the upper body for ailments of the lower body," such as *Hou Chi* (Small Intestine 3 — on the cubital edge of the hand behind the metacarpal-phalangeal articulation of the little finger) for affections of the head and neck; *Yung Ch'uan* (Kidney 1 located at the sole of the foot within the crease formed when the toes are flexed) for cerebral accident, etc. Conversely, use *Pai Hui* (Governing Vessel 20 on the median line of the head, at the parietal eminence in the sagittal line, seven inches above the posterior hairline) for rectal prolapse; *Shui Kou* (Governing Vessel 26 on the median line of the face, below the nose, in the center of the philtrum) for lumbar pain.

(2) Local Point. — By palpation, find the more sensitive or sore spot or spots and then select an acupuncture point nearby. For example, use *Chung Kuan* (Vessel of Conception 12, on the median line of the abdomen four inches above the umbilicus) for stomach spasm, gastritis, etc.; *Shang Hsing* (Governing Vessel 23 on the median line of the cranium one inch inside the frontal hairline) for headache.

(3) Adjacent or Neighboring Points. — Use the points that are adjacent or near the affected site. For instance, for stomach illness, use *Chang Men* (Liver 13, at the tip of the 11th rib); for eye ailment, use *Feng Ch'ih* (Gall Bladder 20, on the posterior surface of the neck, 1.5 inches from the median line, at the height of the point of the mastoid). This method can be used in combination with local points to potentiate the therapeutic effect, or it can be used in place of the local point.

The three methods described above may be employed individually or in combination. For example, for stomach ailment, we may use the distant points *Tsu San Li* (Stomach 36) and *Nei Kuan* (Pericardium 6); local point *Chung Kuan* (Vessel of Conception 12) or *Chang Men* (Liver 13).

VI. Techniques Used in Acupuncture Anesthesia

According to recent reports from Chinese literature, there are certain factors essential for successful induction and maintenance of acupuncture anesthesia.

A. Choice of points. Basically, the spots are selected according to the old classic principle of "following the *ching* (meridian) to pick the spots." To be effective, the needle or needles must be applied at a point or a few points along the *ching* which supposedly runs through the ailing part or organ of the body. In anesthesia, the same principle applies.

B. *Te Ch'i.* It is of utmost importance to attain *Te Ch'i* (acquiring a life-giving or dynamic force) in acupuncture treatment because it is a manifestation of the functioning of *ching lo* (meridians). This means that before the needle can yield any result after its application, the patient must feel sore, distended, heavy and numb over the site of needle placement, and at the same time, the acupuncturist must feel the sensation that the needle in his hand seems to have been slightly "sucked in." As recorded in the classic *Nei Ching*, "to make the needle effective the important thing is *Te Ch'i.*"

C. Adequate induction. An adequate amount of stimulation caused by induction is the key to the success of acupunctural anesthesia. It has been found from experience that a sufficient period (at least 20 minutes) for induction is essential. The inserted needles may be moved and vibrated mechanically by hand or activated electrically. In most cases, the reaction to the needle is directly proportional to the amount of stimulation.

D. Continuous stimulation. To maintain acupunctural anesthesia, it is essential to preserve the sense of *Te Ch'i* by continuous manipulation of the needle.

E. Patient's cooperation with the surgeon. Before the operation, the surgeon should make the patient understand how acupunctural anesthesia is applied, how the operation is carried out, how to perform abdominal breathing (for certain operations such as pneumonectomy) and how he would feel during the operation. With the patient ideologically prepared, the patient can cooperate very well with the surgeon in the course of the operation, and the operation can usually be carried out smoothly.

REFERENCES

Essentials of Chinese Acupuncture (in Chinese) by the Editing Committee on Essentials of Acupuncture, Reprint of 1964 edition, Hong Kong: Ta-Kwan Publ. Co., 1970.

Mann, Felix: *Acupuncture, the Ancient Art of Healing,* 2nd ed., London, W. Heinemann, 1971.

Hung-ch'i (Red Flag), No. 9, August 7, 1971.

Palos, Stephen: *The Chinese Art of Healing,* New York, Herder & Herder, 1971.

Chapter 5

ACUPUNCTURE ANESTHESIA IN THE MODERN CHINESE OPERATING ROOM: PERSONAL OBSERVATIONS

Samuel Rosen

Together with herbal medicines, acupuncture has been used to reduce pain for more than 4000 years. Since 1958, however, with the new emphasis on prevention and service for all the people, the Chinese have been experimenting with acupuncture for anesthetic purposes. Dr. Wu performed his first tonsillectomy using acupuncture anesthesia in 1959 and now has done over 1500 of such procedures with this method of surgical pain prevention.

In the Kwangtung Provincial People's Hospital in Canton the chief of surgery explained to us that his team had carried out over five hundred goiter removals using acupuncture. The Chinese were quick to point out that the method was still imperfect and that about 10 percent of the patients needed conventional anesthesia. During abdominal surgery, especially, some of them complained of pulling sensations during the manipulation of the viscera.

Generally it is up to the prospective patient to decide whether he wants conventional anesthesia or acupuncture. Usually there is a discussion before-hand between the doctor, the patient and his family. In some cases the surgeons themselves decide against the use of acupuncture because they believe that the patient is too nervous or tense. The explanation is that it would be unfair to have a person in such a state consciously go through a major operative procedure. In certain abdominal cases the muscular development of the patient's belly and his inability to relax are also contraindications for the use of acupuncture.

Most of the candidates for surgery receive some opiate derivative such as 50 mg. of Demerol pre-operatively. Moreover, at every operation there is a back-up Western trained anesthesiologist present in the event that the anesthesia induced by acupuncture is insufficient. The acupuncturist, a member of the surgical team, inserts his needles in certain areas of the body previously cleaned with alcohol-soaked sponges. I don't know the reason for their precise implantations at prescribed locations and am not even sure whether the Chinese possess a rationale for their method. In various instances and at different hospitals, I witnessed the use of needles in varying areas for the same surgical procedure. Before we went into the operating room to observe our first case, the surgeon in charge told me that when he first heard about this kind of anesthesia he believed it to be a hoax. Seeing time and again the ensuing anesthetic effects, he finally abandoned his preconceived bias against acupuncture in favor of the obvious evidence of his senses.

At first, after 1958, the Chinese apparently used a large number of acupuncture needles in order to achieve an adequate anesthetic effect. For example, for a total pneumonectomy, they employed about seventy needles but with gradual experience they were able to reduce this number until they now need only one. The acupuncturist generally effortlessly twirls his inserted needles about 120 times a minute. Sometimes the needles placed at various angles are connected to a small battery set which gives off from six to nine volts, especially for longer procedures and when a larger number of twirling needles are required for the achievement of proper anesthesia. Before the first incision was made I stayed close to the head of the operating table, looking intensely at the patient and wondering whether I could detect any changes when the knife started cutting the skin. Time and time again I saw no changes in the expression on the patient's face nor was there any sweating.

The patient's blood pressure was being closely monitored as during any other surgical intervention. I was really quite surprised at the scant amount of bleeding which occurred during the various operations, especially after some long incisions and no spurts of blood. Most bleeding was stopped by the use of clamps.

Acupuncture anesthesia is inexpensive and safe. The Chinese surgeons prefer using it on patients who are in shock, for Caesarean sections and on the aged. Dr. Dudley White witnessed open-heart surgery performed with acupuncture anesthesia. With inhalation anesthesia there is always the possibility of nausea and vomiting and it takes quite a while for homeostasis to return to normal. Such a patient may be in the recovery room for many hours under constant and detailed observation. Many of the patients I observed had sips of tea or milk during and immediately after surgery, and some of them walked out of the operating room under their own power after shaking hands all around. The analgesic effect is said to remain for several hours following surgery. Incidentally, all of the operations which I witnessed were successful. They told me that acupuncture anesthesia had even been employed on 8 month old babies. If I was back in China today, I would like to quiz the patients in more detail and ask them how they feel on their way to and from the operating room. Why do they seem so relaxed without any apparent fear and worry?

I have been privileged to receive a silent motion picture depicting the use of acupuncture anesthesia in cases of major surgery. The film, recently made in the People's Republic, was made available to me by the members of China's delegation to the United States and is extraordinarily impressive. Wherever it has been shown, the movie has left no doubts in the minds of the viewers that they were witnessing a landmark in the conquest of pain during surgery.

It would be nice if someone other than the Chinese was able to duplicate what is now being done in the People's Republic with acupuncture anesthesia. I hope that the time will come soon when we will be able to repeat these procedures here in the U.S. Before we left China we talked with the Revolutionary Committee of the Chinese Medical Association and suggested that American physicians should go to China to learn acupuncture anesthesia as well as Chinese physicians visit our country and demonstrate the method. The authorities seemed very receptive to such an exchange and I believe that it is going to happen, hopefully soon.

Somebody asked whether China could furnish statistics on the comparative results of the use of acupuncture versus general anesthetics. It would be nice if the Chinese did have such figures but in all likelihood these are not available. In the first place, they have only been performing major surgery on a large scale since 1968, nearly close to half a million procedures in all parts of China. Prior to that, the country went through a frightful period of cultural revolution during which everything was chaotic and the schools—colleges and medical schools—were closed. Moreover, there were no scientific publications during the upheaval.

We were told when we left that the schools are once more beginning to open and that soon they would have scientific publications for us. The Chinese will make their statistical analysis of the results of acupuncture anesthesia in due time.

Finally, much experimentation is going on in the People's Republic in search of a neurophysiological explanation of acupuncture anesthesia. When we came out of the hospitals in Canton after witnessing surgery with acupuncture, we asked the surgeon: "Look, all of these patients come into the operating room with Mao's little red book of quotations and they seem to have great confidence in the surgeon. They appear very loyal and composed; don't you think that this may be autosuggestion or autohypnosis?"

The response of our hosts to possible psychosomatic factors operative in acupuncture anesthesia was to point out that they could achieve similar results in young children as well as in animals, such as cats. A more dramatic example was furnished recently to another visiting American biologist and Nobel

Laureate, George Wald. To offset his challenge of a possible hypnotic component in acupuncture anesthesia, his hosts drove him one day to a veterinary school outside of Peking and confronted him with a healthy mule. Then, they shaved the mule's hair off its abdomen, tied the fore and hindlegs down, placed one acupuncture needle in each foreleg and one in each thigh. Subsequently, the hosts scrubbed up and draped the mule as if it were a patient, making a large abdominal incision long enough to pull out a loop of intestine and hold it up for Prof. Wald to photograph. Then, they placed the bowels back in the cavity, closed the incision and untied the mule. The animal calmly got up and had a meal without displaying any signs of discomfort. So, cats and mules know very little about the thought of Mao Tse-Tung to be suggestible unless, as a friend of mine facetiously remarked, in China they can read.

Chapter 6

(ACUPUNCTURE ANESTHESIA)

Nancy Wu

Since the news of China's use of acupuncture to induce anesthesia reached the Western world, the reaction among the general public has been one of surprise and curiosity. But people of the medical profession find the system hard to believe. Many, in fact, regard it as a hoax or think that it probably works through hypnotism. This reaction is to be expected considering the average Westerners' inadequate and often misleading knowledge of medicine in China, which has resulted from the lack of communication between China and the West. This is due in part to the great language barrier which bars Western scientists from examining fairly China's scientific achievements.

Being a physician trained in the Western tradition, it was only recently that I started to develop interest in the study of acupuncture. However, I would like to report on what I have learned from the Chinese literature on the subject with the hope that it may benefit the medical professionals, anesthesiologists in particular. To quote Dr. Nicholas M. Greene's editorial view in Anesthesiology (1), this subject "might just prove to be a potentially valuable contribution to the field of anesthesiology."

The application of acupuncture to anesthesia is a relatively recent venture; its practice has been known in China for thirteen years. Although current medical literature in English is not available due to a suspension of publication, earlier reports on acupuncture anesthesia can be found in the Chinese medical journals of 1959 and 1960 (2-5). These articles reported a technique called electro-acupuncture which was done by first inserting a needle at some points near or distant to the operative sites and

then connecting these needles to an electric device to maintain
a vibrating stimulation. This method of producing analgesia was
applied to dental and oral surgical work including cleft lip repair,
otorhinolaryngalogy and also to some gynecological procedures.
The effect of electro-acupuncture was reported to approach that
of nerve blockage with local anesthetic agents.

Aside from the reports by one of the medical doctors who
recently visited China (6), a general review on the subject of
acupuncture anesthesia is presented in four lengthy articles in
Hung Ch'i (7-10), which discuss the theories of acupuncture
anesthesia. The history of the development of acupuncture
as given in the article "Why surgery can be done under acupuncture anesthesia" tells of many hardships during the early
years. It is stressed that the adaptation of acupuncture to anesthesia was a gradual development. The basis of its origin is the
ancient discovery of the pain-relieving property of acupuncture
plus the extensive clinical experience of the traditional Chinese
medical profession. In 1958 acupuncture was first tried for painful
dressing changes, and was also found to be effective in relieving
sore throat in post-tonsillectomies. These observations led doctors
to think that acupuncture, if applied before surgery, might possibly provide anesthesia for surgery. A trial of acupuncture
anesthesia for tonsillectomy was successful.

During 1960 trials of acupuncture anesthesia were extended
to major operations such as lung resection and many obstacles
were encountered. The goal was finally reached after five years
of struggle and two hundred trial cases. This effort was called
the "first step" in experience working toward the application of
acupuncture anesthesia for other types of operations.

The key to successful pain relief with acupuncture, according
to the reports, is to get a sensation which resembles the description of paresthesia. The sensation of heaviness, soreness, distention and numbness which is designated by the traditional Chinese
medicine as "ch'i" or "vital force" is taken as the end point of acupuncture treatment and elevation of pain threshold at the "related region" can be proven by a "pain measuring device." The
reports say that it was not necessary to insert numerous needles

to provide analgesia for an operation. Prescriptions which had been proposed earlier had required as many as 80 needles. The points of needling were chosen according to the ancient acupuncture charts. These were the points on the meridians which ran across the operative field. But, so many needles were obviously difficult to work with and imposed a great hardship upon the patient. In the next step the most effective points were chosen with the aid of the "pain measuring device," and hundreds of thousands of experiments. An improved technique using just 7 acupuncture needles was proven to be satisfactory for pulmonary resection. But, merely retaining the needle in place after its insertion, as used in the conventional acupuncture technique, would not produce the sustained analgesia necessary for surgery. The needle had to be manipulated constantly either by hand or by an electric device to maintain persistent stimulation and sustained analgesia.

In the district of Shanghai over a period of ten years, 50,000 patients have had operations under acupuncture anesthesia. They ranged from the newborn to people 80 years old, from good risks to those in shock and coma, from those with disease sites in the head, thorax, and abdomen to those with diseased extremities. It is reported that by now 90 percent of the hospitals in Shanghai have adopted this technique of anesthesia.

The statistics compiled during the past ten years and reported in these three articles are listed in Table I. They cover over 200 different types of operations including removal of brain tumors; repair of skull fractures; cataract extraction; tonsillectomies; subtotal thyroidectomies; excision of thyroid tumors and carcinoma of esophagus; cholecystectomies; appendectomies; and other gastro-intestinal operations; lung resection and mitral valve surgery; ovariectomies; laminectomies and operations on the extremities.

The requirements of successful acupuncture anesthesia as stated in these articles are quite pertinent.

1) A pre-operative explanation to the patient concerning the acupuncture and the surgical procedure is essential to allay apprehension and to win the patient's confidence and co-operation.

A nervous patient with increased muscle tension can affect the correctness of needling. This requirement, in fact, tallies with the routine practice of the physician of Western tradition. The surgeons and anesthesiologists regard the pre-operative visits as an integral part of the medical practice.

2) The effect of acupuncture anesthesia normally depends upon a correct placement of the needle with a period of around 20 minutes' inducement.

3) In regard to selecting the sites of needling, the Chinese claim that there are many variations. Tests done on hundreds of thousands of volunteers and numerous "trials" of acupuncture anesthesia on surgical patients show that it is possible to use as little as one or two points to produce the desirable anesthesia. Further studies show that analgesia can be obtained by simply inserting the needle to the nerve which supplies the organ, for instance, cervical plexus for the thyroid operations, or by stimulating the nerve with electrodes without the use of needles. They also show that one needling site can be used for several different operations and either one of the several different acupuncture points, on the ear and on the body, can be used to do the same operation.

It is stressed in these reports that developing positive thinking in both the patient and the medical professionals is helpful to obtain a satisfactory "acupuncture stimulation." In as much as the patient is in a wakeful state during the operative procedure, good coordination between the patient and the physician will reduce or eliminate the discomfort which is elicited from visceral traction. To cope with the operative condition, the patient has to learn to breathe properly and the surgery demands a speedy, steady, accurate and gentle manipulation.

The Chinese have offered some hypotheses to explain their findings and admitted that these hypotheses are far from perfect. However, they have long been convinced that acupuncture works through a neutral pathway and exerts its effects on both central and autonomic nervous systems. (11) The pain relieving mechanism of acupuncture, as they suggested, probably results from "stimulation-inhibition." During acupuncture "stimulation" impulses are transmitted to the brain causing a blockage or inhibition of the cerebral cortex which then does not respond to the painful surgical stimulation. Another suggestion is that this mechanism of "stimulation-inhibition" is probably taking place in the nonspecific reticular system, and at the various levels of the central nervous system. Along with their proposals they reported several interesting clinical and laboratory observations.

1) During the stimulation by acupuncture in patients with normal cortical function, slow waves indicating "inhibition" appeared on EEG tracings. These were not seen in patients with loss of cortical function.

2) In animal experiments acupuncture could erase or lower the evoked potentials resulting from surgical stimulation.

3) The integrity of the nervous conduction is essential in acupuncture anesthesia. Needling the points on limbs paralyzed either through disease or by a local anesthetic block produced no change on the brain wave nor any rise of the pain threshold on the "related regions." However, changes were observed when the unaffected limb was stimulated by acupuncture.

4) Acupuncture has effect on the autonomic nervous system:

a) There were increases in circulation time, red cells, white cells, and blood sugar tested two hours after acupuncture. However, these changes did not occur in patients with interrupted nervous conduction.

b) In some other instances changes in skin temperature and blood pressure were observed. The latter was illustrated by two cases: In one, a patient who was hypotensive due to an empyema of the gall bladder, had his blood pressure return to normal after acupuncture. In the other, a patient who was hypertensive for years came in for an appendectomy; acupuncture lowered his blood pressure incidentally. These instances were regarded as beneficiary by-products of acupuncture.

5) In researching the anatomical structural relations of the 365 acupuncture points on the body, it was found that about one-half of the points are directly above the peripheral nerves and the other half are a few millimeters from the nerves.

In recent years the scientists' concepts of the mechanism of pain have entered a new stage. (12-13) Such modern concepts, though still somewhat controversial (14), are supported by experimental findings and clinical observations (15-22), and are helpful for interpretation on many empiric experiences. With the new concept, it is possible to explain how acupuncture interrupts the pain pathways and such a view has been expressed by many Western physicians. The effects of acupuncture as reported are quite complex. This is to be expected if acupuncture exerts its effects on such intricate machinery as the nervous system.

The history of modern anesthesia in the West is only a little over a hundred years old. Scientists have been searching for an ideal anesthetic agent that possesses anesthetic potency and all other desirable qualities but is free of deleterious effects on the cardiovascular and respiratory functions. To date not one of the anesthetics used fulfills all of the requirements. Anesthetics may affect every system in the body and the effects may linger on during the post-operative period prolonging the duration of convalescence. Such complications as prolonged narcosis, nausea, and vomiting, airway obstruction and respiratory depression are common. To cope with the requirements of the surgery and the individual patient, anesthesiologists choose different techniques and combinations of anesthetic agents, in order to minimize the untoward effects of anesthesia on bodily functions. Rapid development of the science of anesthesia during the last few decades has enhanced the growth of sophisticated surgery and has enabled surgeons to even perform difficult operations on poor-risk patients. However, there are patients who cannot tolerate anesthesia, because of their disturbed cardiovascular and respiratory functions. Moreover, some patients who have inborn defects, develop fatal reactions such as malignant hyperthermia from anesthetic agents. Under certain circumstances there are distinct advantages in having the patient remain conscious for procedures such as plastic repairs to retain his muscle tone and voluntary movements in order to evaluate the operative results. The limitations of local and regional anesthesia with local anesthetic drugs are well known. Its conduct cannot meet many surgical requirements, and is unsuitable for sensitive and tense patients. However, a good pre-operative explanation and pre-anesthetic medication can often put the patient at ease, while at times light general anesthesia is used in conjunction with regional anesthesia to allay apprehension.

We shall await for more data on the precise technique, the indications and contraindications, the incidence of failure, and above all, the complications in China's new development. Hopefully, direct communication and an exchange of scientists will bring about firsthand information, allowing us to soon find out whether or not this technique can be adapted to our practice of anesthesiology.

TABLE I

(The statistics are taken from the publication HUNG-CH'I (Red Flag) No. 9, 1971)

Hospital	No. of Cases	Success rate
Hospitals in the District of Shanghai	50,000	90%
People's Liberation Army General	10,000	90%
General Hospital of People's Liberation Army Units in Canton	13,000	96.4%

REFERENCES

1. Green, N. M.: "This is no humbug — or is it?" — Editorial View, *Anesthesiol.* 36 (1972), 101.
2. "Anesthetization by electro-acupuncture upon nerve and clinical application of electro-needling anesthesia," *Chinese Journal of Surgery* (in Chinese) 7 (1959), 453-457. Abstract (in English) *Chinese Med. J.* 78 (1959), 586.
3. Yeh, J. H.: "Electro-acupuncture in place of anesthesia in obstetrics and gynecology," *Chinese Journal of Obstetrics and Gynecology* (in Chinese) 7 (1959), 397. Abstract (in English) *Chinese Med. J.* 79 (1959), 559.
4. Sheng, L. C. and Chang, T. H.: "Electro-acupuncture anesthesia in oral surgery," *Chinese Med. J.* 80 (1960), 97-99.
5. Chao, Po-hsueh: "Acupuncture anesthesia in E.N.T. operations," *Chinese J. of Otorhinolaryngology* (in Chinese) 8 (1960), 115. Abstract (in English) *Chinese Med. J.* 80 (1960), 398-399.

6. Dimond, E. G.: "Medical education and care in China," *J.A.M.A.* 218 (1971), 1558-1583.

7. Shanghai Cooperative Group of Acupuncture Anesthesia, "Why surgery can be done under acupuncture anesthesia," *Hung Ch'i* (in Chinese) 9 (1971), 59.

8. General Hospital of the People's Liberation Army Report, "Some knowledge regarding the theory of acupuncture anesthesia," *Hung Ch'i* (in Chinese) 9 (1971), 70.

9. Kwangchow General Hospital of the People's Liberation Army Units, Report, "Investigation into the theory of pain relieving property of acupuncture," *Hung Ch'i* (in Chinese) 9 (1971), 75.

10. Peking Cooperative Group of Acupuncture Anesthesia, "Acupuncture points, meridians and the theory of acupuncture anesthesia," *Hung Ch'i* (in Chinese) 12 (1971), 63.

11. Chu, Lien: *Hsin Chên-Chiu-hsüeh* (Textbook of Modern Acupuncture and Moxibustion), Public Health Press: Peking, 1956.

12. Melzack, R. and Wall, P. D.: "Pain mechanisms: a new theory," *Science* 150 (1965), 971-979.

13. Waltz, T. A. and Ehni, G.: "The thalamic syndrome and its mechanism," *Neurosurg.* 24 (1966), 735-742.

14. Vyklicky, L., et al.: "Primary afferent depolarization evoked by a painful stimulus," *Science* 165 (1969), 184.

15. Shealy, C. N.: "The physiological substrate of pain," *Headache* 6 (1966), 101-108.

16. Wall, P. D. and Sweet, W. H.: "Temporary abolition of pain in man," *Science* 155 (1967), 108-109.

17. Sweet, W. H. and Wepsic, J. G.: "Treatment of chronic pain by stimulation of fibers of primary afferent neuron," *Transactions of the American Neurological Association* 93 (1968), 103-107.

18. Shealy, C. N., Taslitz, N., Mortimer, J. T., and Becker, D. P.: "Electrical inhibition of pain: experimental evaluation," *Anesth. Analg. Cur. Res.* 46 (1969), 299-305.

19. Shealy, C. N., Mortimer, J. T., and Reswick, J. B.: "Electrical inhibition of pain by stimulation of the dorsal columns: preliminary clinical report," *Anesth. Analg. Cur. Res.* 46 (1967), 489-491.

20. Shealy, C. N.: "Dorsal column electro-analgesia," *J. Neurosurg.* 32 (1970), 560.

21. Higgins, J. D., Tursky, B., and Schwarts, G. E.: "Shock-elicited pain and its reduction by concurrent tactile stimulation," *Science* 172 (1971), 866-867.

22. Fellner, C. H.: "Alteration in pain perception under conditions of multiple sensory modality stimulation," *Psychosomatics* 12 (1971), 313-315.

Chapter 7

(ACUPUNCTURAL ANESTHESIA)

Removal of Lung under Acupuncture Anesthesia
(edited version)

Report from Peking, December 28, 1971 in
Survey of China Mainland Press, Jan., 1972

Acupuncture anesthesia is a unique method created by Chinese medical workers to develop a Chinese medical legacy and combine western and traditional Chinese medicine. I watched a pneumonectomy at the Peking Tuberculosis Research Institute recently, and saw the wonder performed by a small needle.

One of the biggest of its kind in China, the Research Institute in Tunghsien County on the outskirts of Peking has more than 400 beds. Everything was ready for the operation when I arrived at the operating room around nine that morning. Shortly thereafter, the patient walked into the room accompanied by nurses. Li Tsui-hsia, a twenty-four year old primary school teacher from northeast China, was suffering from multiple tuberculous cavities of the right lung which necessitated its complete removal. The doctors greeted her warmly and asked:

"Did you sleep well?"

"I did."

"Do you feel nervous?"

"No," the patient answered with a smile, looking very calm. She lay down on the operating table, and an anesthetist named Fu Chung-li took a small needle and inserted it at an acupuncture point in the outer aspect of the patient's right forearm. As he twirled the needle he asked her how she felt. "I feel something like distention in my arm," she replied. This indicated that the needling had begun to induce analgesia. The twirling continued for another twenty minutes and then the patient was ready for surgery.

Hsin Yu-ling, the surgeon in charge, is highly experienced. Now in his fifties, he joined the Eighth Route Army during the war of resistance again Japanese aggression when he was a teenager and worked as a medical orderly. His two assistants for this operation were very young, one standing beside him and the other facing him. The anesthetist sat behind the head of the patient and kept twirling the needle. A medical assistant recorded the blood pressure and pulse. One nurse handed the surgeons the various instruments and another took charge of transfusions and infusions.

After sterilizing the patient's chest and back, the surgeons injected some saline and adrenalin into the portion of the chest to be operated on. The saline, they said, would facilitate the incision and the adrenalin would alleviate hemorrhage. They also injected 0.2 mg. of Luminal, 10 mg. of morphine and 0.3 mg. of atropine. These drugs which would produce only a mild sedative effect and help reduce the secretion of the mucosa of the respiratory tract (patients with T.B. generally discharge much sputum), were used as pre-anesthetic medication. Analgesia was to be produced mainly by needling, while the small amount of pre-anesthetic medication would alleviate the patient's anxiety and reduce exhaustion.

The surgeons commented that some people in medical circles once insisted that no medicine should be used in the course of acupuncture anesthesia. Now most of the medical workers have agreed that in developing ancient Chinese acupuncture, or, specifically, in applying acupuncture anesthesia, attention should be paid to the advantages of Western medicine and pharmacology and to combining Western and traditional Chinese medicine so as to create new medicine and pharmacology. The fact that both traditional Chinese doctors and Western doctors worked at the same operating table was a manifestation of the combination of both types of medicine.

After the skin was incised at 10:15 a.m., the anesthetist asked the patient: "The operation has begun, how do you feel?"

"No pain," the patient answered calmly. The surgeons remarked that the skin is most sensitive and if the incision does not cause pain, then the acupuncture anesthesia has been initially successful. The surgeons went ahead systematically, accurately and quickly to open the chest.

Again the anesthetist, Dr. Fu, asked the patient how she felt. She said that she was having some difficulty breathing, which is natural when the right lung is collapsed by the air entering the chest. Dr. Fu advised her to inhale deeply. The patient carried out his instructions ventilating slowly and evenly from the abdomen. Some patients feel uncomfortable from visceral traction. Deep breathing helps resist stimulation from the operation and eases the feeling of respiratory embarrassment. A few minutes passed. Once again the doctor asked the patient how she felt and she responded that she could now breathe more easily.

Dr. Fu was trained in traditional Chinese medicine. He started learning acupuncture anesthesia in 1965 and has since performed numerous operations. During this operation he twirled the needle with either hand in turn, in an even rhythm. Now and then he whispered to the patient what point the operation had reached and what she should do. Patient and doctor cooperated well.

Each time acupuncture anesthesia is used, the patient is fully informed beforehand of the procedures and the contingencies, as well as what he or she may feel during the operation. In cases of pulmonary resection, the patients are taught abdominal breathing. This prepares them to cooperate with the surgeons and is important in ensuring the proper anesthetic effect. The use of acupuncture anesthesia which keeps the patient conscious makes active cooperation between patient and surgeon possible in such major operations.

The operation proceeded smoothly. The patient's blood pressure, pulse and breathing remained stable and the diseased lung was removed. When the doctor told her this, the patient was surprised and greatly pleased. Speedily and carefully, the surgeons stitched up the incision. The patient remained calm and informed Dr. Fu that she was hungry. A nurse fed her some pieces of orange as the surgeons continued.

At 12:15 p.m. the operation was completed. The doctors helped the patient sit up. She was in a good mood and told the surgeons she had not felt any pain during the operation, except some difficulty in breathing at certain stages of the procedure. The volume of her voice was almost as loud as before surgery. She was returned to her ward.

Patients undergoing chest operations usually receive general anesthesia, and after the operation the patient remains unconscious for several hours. Acupuncture anesthesia helps the patient move about, take food early and recover more quickly. The patient does not suffer from any headache, nausea, or other unfavorable side-reactions. An increasing number of patients today prefer this method. By the end of 1970, acupuncture anesthesia had been used in 400,000 operations.

I warmly congratulated the medical workers on their success. They expressed their firm determination to make continued progress, constantly sum up their experiences, improve their methods as well as do their share in mastering medical science.

Chapter 8

SOME KNOWLEDGE REGARDING THE THEORY OF ACUPUNCTURE ANESTHESIA

A Report of the Chinese People's Liberation
Army General Hospital

Free Translation By Nancy Wu

IN RECENT YEARS, based on learning from the experiences of fraternal hospitals, we have performed surgery under acupuncture anesthesia. All together, 200 different types of operations were performed, and over 10,000 cases were treated with a success rate of more than 90 percent. This large amount of practical application shows that acupuncture anesthesia is safe, effective, convenient, and economical. It can shorten a patient's convalescence, be made widely available in the Army Corps and the rural areas, and is especially suited to the needs of emergency wartime conditions. Now, in order to sum up the rich experience of acupuncture anesthesia, promote a rise from intuitive feeling to rational understanding and develop further techniques of acupuncture anesthesia, we raise some preliminary views concerning the principles of acupuncture anesthesia.

Adequate "stimulating quantity": key to success in acupuncture anesthesia

"Stimulating quantity" is a concept that has been gradually formulated during our clinical practice. During our early development of acupuncture anesthesia, we prescribed using numerous acupuncture points. Then, after prescribing so many points, the question became, just which is the best one to adopt? Is the success of acupuncture anesthesia dependent upon such numerous prescriptions? We have gone through different types of experiments comparing and contrasting them over and over in an attempt to reduce the number of points. Some studies were done by self experimentation, and from dozens of points related to the eye, just two points were selected for cataract operations. The anesthetic effect was satisfactory. Some studies were done by case analysis, with one set of prescriptions being chosen from ten different ones designed for tubal ligation. Again, the operation was successful. Some applied the same point to different operations, others adopted different points for the same operation. All these practical applications enabled us to realize that since in the practice of acupuncture anesthesia, variabilities of points can be great, the make-up of the prescription was not the key to success. Secondly the wide variance in type and method of acupuncture anesthesia for surgery came to our attention. We saw that needles could be inserted in the body, or in the ear, that they could be manipulated by hand or activated by an electric device, or that the points could be blocked off, all with little difference in the anesthetic effect. This showed that the type and method of acupuncture anesthesia were not the key to success either. Our clinical practice did prove though, that no matter what the prescription of points, or the type and method of application, it must have a sufficient time for inducement. If the inducement period is too short, the analgesic effect is poor; by extending the inducement period to a definite degree a good analgesic effect can be obtained. This inducement is "the production through needling of a sensation of soreness, numbness, distention and heaviness, that is "a gaining of the vital force (*ch'i*)." When the stimulation reaches a certain quantity, the analgesic effect is produced. Consequently, we believe that building up an adequate amount of stimulation through inducement is the key to success in acupuncture anesthesia.

After we have formulated the concept of *"stimulating quantity"* we can better understand the structural correlation of the location, the method, and the time of the stimulation, and their role in the acupuncture anesthesia. We can thus boldly simplify the selection of acupuncture points and prescriptions by choosing one or several of the more sensitive points on the body and then perform the surgical operation. For instance, we have used only a single point to successfully perform operations on different locations of the body, such as lobectomies, excision of pterygium, and appendectomy; we have also used one pair of points to produce anesthesia for such major operations as gastric, bowel, and ovarian cyst resections. But, it has been proven from practice that, regardless of whether we needle the body, ear, face or nose, a successful acupuncture anesthesia can be obtained only if the selected points and the method of manipulation can guarantee the patient an adequate quantity of stimulation.

With this understanding, we proceeded to work on the method of stimulation so as to raise its quantity and thereby strengthen the effect of acupuncture anesthesia. To make the patient "gain *ch'i*" is the most important process of acupuncture anesthesia; without such a sensation, no matter how many needles are used or how long the needles are twirled, it is to no avail. Such unresolved problems of acupuncture anesthesia as incomplete analgesia, muscle tension, and visceral traction reflex, are related to the technique of manipulating the needle. We realize that when using identical prescription of points, if the procedure is not carried out skillfully the muscular tension becomes more pronounced; when the skill is improved, there is no difficulty in closing the abdominal incision, and the visceral traction reflex is also not apparent. This shows that the skill is an important requirement for obtaining stimulating quantity. During the time of stimulation, not only do we emphasize the preoperative inducement but also for those long, major operations, if twirling of the needles has been stopped for quite a while intraoperatively, they should be twirled again before the closure of the abdominal or chest incisions.

Just how much stimulating quantity is considered "adequate" differs because of the various effects of different surgical procedures upon the patient and individual variations in patient tolerance. Generally, it depends upon the type and duration of operation and the degree of the patient's reaction to the needling sensation. In most cases, the needling sensation is directly proportional to the stimulating quantity. Before an adequate stimulation is obtained, an increase in quantity will improve the efficiency of the acupuncture anesthesia, but one cannot generalize and say that the greater the stimulating quantity the better the efficiency of acupuncture anesthesia.

From Concept of Stimulating Quantity to Hypothesizing a Theory of Acupuncture Anesthesia

To further improve the effectiveness of acupuncture anesthesia, one must explore and grasp the characteristics of the antagonism between the acupuncture analgesia and the surgical pain, that is, we must understand in what part of the body, through what kind of structures and how, does the antagonism take place.

Since acupuncture anesthesia is developed from the traditional Chinese acupuncture, seeking the theory of acupuncture anesthesia will naturally involve the problems of meridians. Concerning this problem our thoughts are: first, the meridian system is a concept formulated by traditional Chinese medicine over a long period of clinical and therapeutical practice based on the relations between the diagnosis and treatment of diseases. The acupuncture points of the entire body have been classified and unified. To a definite degree, it shows the laws of correlation between different parts of the organism, and also explains pathological and physiological processes. To treat disease and to alleviate pain, acupuncture mainly exerts its effects through the regulation of meridians, which includes the regulation of functions of the nervous system and the body fluid. Acupuncture anesthesia is intended for surgery and for alleviating pain; although the evidence of regulation also occurs during the procedure of acupuncture anesthesia, it is not its main function. Second, the meridian theory was formulated mainly by summarizing the clinical practice and due to limitations of the ancient historical conditions, detailed anatomical investigations could not be carried out.

Furthermore, modern anatomical and histological studies have not found an independent meridian system. However, a comparison of meridians with the distribution of the nervous system shows that half of the points are distributed on the nerve trunks. Therefore, we believe the principle of acupuncture anesthesia can be more clearly explained through the function of the nervous system.

Starting from this point of view, we may think that the analgesic effect of acupuncture anesthesia is taking place in the central nervous system. Pain is a sensation. It possesses a physical basis. Its physical basis is the nervous system. Sensation (including pain) is the reflection of the human brain toward the action of objective surroundings. Pain produced by surgery that is the neural impulse (bioelectrical change) resulting from a surgical wound reaches the brain by way of neural transmission and induces a painful sensation. Originally, the fact that needling the points on the body can reduce or relieve pain in certain diseases inspired the development of acupuncture anesthesia. Needling a certain point produces a reaction of soreness, numbness, distention and heaviness. This is also a sensation. The transmission of the neural impulse can not be sensed, but the reaction to the needling through whatever pathway it may travel, eventually reaches the brain where a reflection is shown. Animal experimentations have proved that bioelectrical activities can be recorded from different surfaces and localities of the brain following stimulations both from surgical trauma and acupuncture. Consequently, the central nervous system is the site of analgesic action of acupuncture anesthesia.

During the process of producing pain, there is a transitional change of a quantitative one to a qualitative one. The amount of stimulation required to produce painful reflection is called, in medical terms, pain threshold. We suppose that the stimulating quantity representing the threshold shows how strong a stimulation is received per unit of time, that is the quantity of stimulation equals time multiplied by the intensity of stimulation. This can help us explain a general phenomenon of why under acupuncture anesthesia, better analgesic effect is obtained when a fast incision is made with a sharp knife rather than a slow incision. Acupuncture anesthesia can raise the pain threshold, but the skin incision is a strong stimulation. If the stimulation from the skin incision is prolonged, then its stimulating quantity is greater than the pain threshold, and it can still produce painful reaction. On the other hand, a sharp knife and fast incision shorten the duration of incisional stimulation. Its stimulating quantity then is lesser than the pain threshold, and consequently no pain is felt. Nevertheless, acupuncture anesthesia also gives the patient a considerable amount of stimulating quantity. Why, then, does it not cause pain? This is because the intensity of stimulation from the needling twirled by hand or electric device is low and the stimulating quantity per unit of time is smaller than the pain threshold, therefore it is painless. This explains the relationship between the pain threshold and the stimulating quantity.

That acupuncture anesthesia can raise the pain threshold is an acknowledged fact. How does it work? It is the key question to the principle of acupuncture anesthesia. Some people explain it with the theory of "stimulation-inhibition," believing that the stimulating quantity of acupuncture anesthesia which is smaller than the pain threshold, produces a point of excitation on the cerebral cortex. With the summation of the stimulating quantity, it results in an inhibition around the point of excitation. To arouse the suppressed cortex then requires a greater than normal stimulating quantity. Thus the pain threshold has been raised. This is a fundamental interpretation. We believe that by applying the concept of stimulating quantity, we can proceed further investigating the pain relief of acupuncture anesthesia.

The antagonism of pain and pain-relieving on the body surface is the conflict between the stimulating quantity of the surgical wound and that of the acupuncture anesthesia. Both of these stimuli can generate bioelectricity in the body, which is transmitted through the neural pathway and reaches the brain. In the brain cells it becomes a conflict between the evoked potentials from the surgical wound and that from the acupuncture anesthesia. This phenomenon has been verified by animal experimentations. But how do the bioelectrical currents interact? This is still unclear. We hypothesize three possible conditions:

1) "Strong and weak relationship": a strong bioelectric current inhibits or interferes with a weak one. Acupuncture causes changes of the electrical potential in the tissue structure of the brain cells. The stimulation from the surgical wound must have an even greater stimulating quantity in order to change the electrical potential, thus the pain threshold is raised.

2) "One who enters first is the master": The procedure of acupuncture anesthesia always has to start with manipulating the needle for inducement; analgesia is then obtained for surgical incision. This explains the interaction of bioelectric currents. Not only is there a strong and weak relationship, but also the characteristic of who enters first rejecting those who arrive later. When the brain cells have already been stimulated by acupuncture anesthesia, the late arriving stimulation of the surgical trauma, no matter how strong, will not affect the brain cells. This can also explain why the small stimulation from acupuncture can overcome the strong one of the surgical trauma.

3) "Occupying a superior position": The conflict between the evoked potential of acupuncture and surgical trauma and the number of pain related brain cells, also directly influences the analgesic effect. The function of the inducement period of acupuncture anesthesia is dependent upon "priority is the master" and occupation of a greater number of pain-related brain cells. In view of the fact that the analgesic effect of acupuncture anesthesia is at times incomplete, we believe the bioelectrical activity of "strong overcomes weak" "preoccupation" and "superiority" may exist concurrently.

Developing "Two Positive Thinking," An Even Better Stimulating Quantity is Then Secured

Adequate stimulating quantity is the key to acupuncture anesthesia. To guarantee an adequate amount of stimulating quantity we must mobilize positive thinking in both the medical workers and patient.

With surgery done under acupuncture anesthesia, the patient is in a completely conscious state. The effect of acupuncture anesthesia is not dependent upon the patient's subjective will nor his way of thinking. The psychological factor apparently does not affect the patient's physiological function nor his power to resist the surgical trauma. For instance, increased muscular tension due to anxiety, prevents "gaining *ch'i*" from acupuncture, and as a consequence adequate stimulating quantity can not be obtained. When visceral traction reflex occurs, if the patient can coordinate motions with the surgeon, breathing slowly and deeply for example, the surgical stimulation can be reduced. Therefore, a painstaking and careful preoperative mental preparation designed to fully mobilize the patient's positive thinking is the important link for increasing the efficacy of acupuncture anesthesia.

External factors are variable. With only the patient's positive thinking and not that of the medical personnel, the acupuncture anesthesia will not succeed. The medical workers must worry the patient's worry and sense the patient's sensation. The acupuncturist must conscientiously select the stimulating site and adopt the appropriate method to guarantee the patient adequate stimulating quantity. The surgical personnel must actively cooperate, adopt a gentle, speedy, steady and precise method of manipulation to reduce the surgical trauma. An improvement of surgical manipulation can reduce the stimulating quantity of surgical trauma and thus strengthen the analgesic effect of acupuncture anesthesia. Therefore, to make the acupuncture anesthesia successful, we must fully mobilize positive thinking in both the patient and the medical personnel.

Although we now have some understanding regarding the principle of acupuncture anesthesia, it is a preliminary one and may very well be inaccurate. Further analysis and discussion are required to study the mechanism in depth and to perfect the technique of acupuncture anesthesia.

Chapter 9

A PHYSIOLOGICAL BASIS FOR ELECTRO-ACUPUNCTURE

C. Norman Shealy

I HAVE BEEN INTERESTED in acupuncture for a number of years because it has seemed to me that any technique which has achieved success for thousands of years is bound to have some degree of truth to it. Fortunately, I do not have to attempt an explanation of all the phenomena of acupuncture. These have already been widely discussed and it is generally conceded that Western science is having great difficulty coming to grips with concepts so foreign to our own methods of investigation. Therefore, it should be just as difficult to understand why acupuncture, practiced for thousands of years, has suddenly become so fantastically interesting to the United States, just after minimal political thawing of relations with China. For over twenty years we managed mysteriously to ignore a third of the world's people. Now, suddenly and ironically, we are mesmerized by their most ancient form of medicine.

Prior to this, Americans never had taken advantage of knowledge available to them before 1940 in China nor since then in many European countries. It appears probable that electro-acupuncture, now widely used in the People's Republic to achieve anesthesia, provided the catalyst to spark American interest. Electronics and electricity offer some semblance to known science; thus, the incorporation of electrical current into acupuncture allows the Western mind to think seriously about it without having to acknowledge embarrassment at the previously expressed ignorance and even indifference.

Perhaps most fascinating is the report that electro-acupuncture began to be used only ten years ago, since a paper published in *Science* seven years ago provided the groundwork for the discussion now widely in progress to explain the effects of electro-acupuncture. Indeed, I also was initially inclined to accept Melzack and Wall's "gate" as the mechanism whereby anesthesia might be achieved. The "gate" theory, however, can comfortably accommodate *only local anesthesia;* it does not provide a convenient explanation for pain suppression in areas quite remote from the external electrical stimulus.

Because of our interest in methods of controlling pain, several clinical observations provided us, over six years ago, with an opportunity to begin an investigation of such remote influences. Suffice it to say that I did not originally look upon them as relatives of acupuncture.

Patients complaining of pain often mention a "feeling" of numbness in the offending area. Usually our crude clinical tests with a wisp of cotton or a safety pin do not demonstrate "numbness," and therefore we dismiss the complaint. However, if we find numbness in such tests, it often does not conform to our anatomical concepts of dermatomal distribution and the patient is then commonly labeled hysterical. Patients such as this, even with clear-cut organic problems, are summarily sent to psychiatrists.

If we examine such patients closely we learn that the "numbness" is rarely total or severe, although occasionally it may be complete enough to produce anesthesia. The anatomical distribution of the complaint is rather interesting. It commonly involves one leg, with or without the ipsilateral arm; or one arm. Occasionally, the numbness involves half the face and/or the head; rarely involving an entire half of the body. *The phenomenon practically never occurs in the absence of pain.*

In such a patient, if we search carefully for trigger areas such as small focal regions of exquisite tenderness, we are usually rewarded. Furthermore, pressure on such trigger points elicits not only local pain, but usually evokes pain spreading far from the trigger site. Often patients feel increased numbness in the affected regions. Local infiltration of the trigger spot with lido-caine, or any other local anesthetic, will relieve not only the focal tenderness but also the referred or reflex pain and numbness. Occasionally, we have found that simple insertion of a needle into the trigger area relieves symptoms, just as a thalamic elec-trode may block, temporarily, Parkinsonism. Almost invariably subpainful electrical current accomplishes the same effect with results lasting, as with a chemical block, from one hour to several days.

In patients with demonstrable physical abnormalities, such as ruptured spinal discs, correction of the pathology leads to immediate clearing of the peculiar numbness. Indeed, there is now excellent evidence that pain of almost the entire disc-syndrome comes not from spinal nerve root compression, but rather from adjacent joints which are anatomically stressed by narrowed disc spaces. Needling of the disc space is not painful; needling the affected facet clearly evokes the clinical pain and numbness, often on the side *opposite* the pathology.

Such clinical evidence, presented in hundreds of patients, must either convince one that the symptoms are real or that one should become a psychiatrist. I personally prefer to accept the symptoms as real.

Therefore, we must seek a physiological system which allows such interactions. In this search we have investigated the effects of physical and electrical stimulation upon a primitive central nervous system pathway in the spinal cord of cats and monkeys. Cells in this polysynaptic pathway are excited or inhibited by almost every input to the body. They fire in a reproducible way to painful stimuli and with different patterns and time courses to both painful and less painful stimuli. They are discharged by touch, vibration, heat, cold, pain and by both non-painful and painful electrical stimuli. At first, we investigated the effects of peripheral stimulation only at spinal or brain sites cephalad to the input and we found strong representation contralaterally as well as ipsilaterally.

Later, we found extensive caudal projections again repre-sented both contralaterally and ipsilaterally. Of particular interest is the relationship of these projections to the head. Electrical stimulation of any part of arms, body or legs is transmitted throughout the entire core of the spinal cord (and brain) in all directions. Stimulation of the head, however, almost never excites this massive pathway *caudal* to the upper cervical area. The striking relationship between head and arm input is reminiscent of many clinical states.

Now we must consider the total capability of the system under discussion. Since it is a multi-modal system with tremendous interneuronal connections, a little goes a long way—perhaps the last place where this is true in today's world! Once a cell is maximally discharging, it cannot accept additional stimuli. Thus, if a cell important to transmission of pain is being fired by touch, vibration, heat, or non-painful electrical stimulation, it is not available for participation in pain. Inhibition of pain requires, then, only that the cells be adequately busy to prevent their activation by a new stimulus. This has been found to be true, both experimentally and clinically. Single stimuli have minimal effect upon this central network; repetitive stimuli, even of a non-painful nature, are additive and gradually evoke the maximum response of which the cells are collectively capable. At this point there is no firing by the addition of pain. The important points here are:

1. This is not a cortical, brain or "emotional" distraction. The same physiological events occur in high spinal or decorticate animals.

2. It is essential that *adequate* non-painful stimulation be applied to the most satisfactory body area. It is difficult, for instance, to inhibit the response to foot pain with concomitant non-painful stimulation only of the foot. Concomitant stimulation of totally unrelated areas, such as the perineal region, may accomplish complete suppression of the response to foot pain. Although we have not exhaustively investigated all acupuncture sites (this would require several lifetimes), certain prime points have been studied. The ulnar and median nerves, approached either directly or through needles which stimulate branches in the mid-forearm, provide extremely potent areas for activation of

the central core. Tongue and ear stimulation also feed into the same cervical regions, although without the caudal representations of their arm associates.

It becomes easier now to understand how the electrical stimulation of ears and forearms is capable of providing anesthesia for abdominal surgery, whereas stimulation of at least some additional cranial area, such as that of the occipital nerve, is required for control of head pain. Although the "gate" is undoubtedly involved in the electrical control of pain, this theory is not the complete answer. The ubiquitous nature of the multimodal spinal network must also be an important part of this mechanism.

About seven years ago, during our investigation into the physiology of pain, we began placing standard surgical or injection type needles into the skin of patients and noted that indeed we could administer local anesthesia as easily with an electrical stimulus as with novocaine. Obviously the former is a much safer method and to my knowledge electro-anesthesia has never damaged the body as a whole. Even the passage of fine needles through the nerves themselves causes no damage.

Our clinical use of this knowledge has led to the application of electrical stimuli to almost all parts of the body. When the pain is localized we first try electrical stimulation of the affected region, but this occasionally accentuates the pain. Then, we stimulate areas surrounding the painful part or we stimulate through needles inserted into the area. If this does not succeed, we resort to electrical stimulation of numerous unrelated regions. Clinically, this method becomes an elaborate project but it often is successful.

This is not the forum for a detailed discussion of clinical results. However, it is worth noting that relief of many pains can be accomplished safely through the application of non-painful electrical stimulation. We have found it especially useful in acute sprains, causalgia, headache, and labor. Indeed, I think that over 75 percent of deliveries will be performed under electro-anesthesia within the next decade. When one cannot adequately control the spinal cord's transmission of pain with external stimulation, it is feasible—and I have done it—to insert through a needle a stimulating electrode intraspinally adjusting it to the proper area to produce abdominal or chest anesthesia.

The spinal cord, the major area of inter-reaction for the entire body, lies between fibers that produce pain—those that carry pain and those that do not. In applying electrical stimulation to the back portion of the spinal cord—the so-called dorsal region—we can effect a relief of pain in approximately 85 percent of our cases. Such a spinal electrode could be left in site for several days to allow excellent control of post-operative pain, without employing the inhibiting mental and physical effects of narcotics.

A fascinating part of this procedure is that pain relief commonly lasts for hours after stimulation. We have patients who have had pain supposedly for 24 hours a day up to seven years. prior to stimulation of the dorsal column of the spinal cord, who can achieve total control of their pain by stimulation of the dorsal column for as little as two minutes out of every 48 hours.

Primarily through external stimulation, all of my chronic patients today receive a tremendous amount of stimulation electrically through the skin and at the present time we are doing some minor surgery with this form of anesthesia. A finger or toe can very easily and safely be amputated under electro-anesthesia. Recently I successfully operated on a man who needed to have the ulnar nerve transplanted. Performed earlier, painless mobilization would also offer an ideal method of rehabilitation. Although electro-acupuncture is still in its infancy, it may become a most potent and valuable therapeutic tool in the current decade. If we use it well, it could be perfected to serve us in ways still unknown.

In summary, the core of the spinal cord contains multimodal cells which respond to almost all sensory stimulation and are initially involved in pain transmission. They project both proximally and distally and if adequately activated by non-painful electrical stimulation, they are unavailable for pain, which must use the same network. Although other physiological changes may be induced through this pathway, our evidence is only sufficient to explain inhibition of pain, either focally or remotely. Such inhibition accomplished by a competitive excitation may be accomplished by physiological inhibition through the "spinal gate" of Melzack and Wall. However, the gate alone does not explain the physiological or the clinical observations mentioned above. Yet, electrical stimulation, carried out transcutaneously, percutaneously, or intraspinally offers an exciting new dimension in the control of pain; and electro-acupuncture is the most dramatic example of such a technique.

REFERENCES

Melzack, R. and Wall, P. D.: "Pain mechanisms: a new theory," *Science* 150 (1965) 971-979.

Shealy, C. N.: "The physiological substrate of pain," *Headache* 6 (1966), 101-108.

Shealy, C. N., Taslitz, N., and Mortimer, J. T.: "Electrical inhibition of pain: experimental evaluation," *Anesth. Analg.* 46 (1967), 299-305.

Shealy, C. N., Mortimer, J. T., and Reswick, J. B.: "Electrical inhibition of pain by stimulation of the dorsal columns: preliminary clinical report," *Anesth. Analg.* 46 (1967), 489-491.

Shealy, C. N.: "Dorsal column electroanalgesia," *J. Neurosurgery* 32 (1970), 560.

PART IV
HEALTH CARE DELIVERY IN MODERN CHINA

Chapter 10

(INTRODUCTION)

Guenter B. Risse

In medical and health work, put the stress on the rural areas.
—Mao Tse-tung
(Directive, June 26, 1965)

AFTER READING AND HEARING the various accounts of those travelers privileged to recently visit the People's Republic of China, one theme seemed to be reoccurring in their narratives: the rather dramatic changes which have taken place in the delivery of health care since the early 1950's. For the first time in China's venerable history a strong central government has been gradually able to provide medical services to the rural population comprising more than two-thirds of the people presently living on the mainland.

Such a monumental achievement, consolidated by the recent Cultural Revolution, deserves our attention and should be studied in more detail in the months and years ahead. Although the practice of acupuncture — especially for surgical analgesia — has caught the interest of the American public, the Chinese view with greater pride their accomplishments in the field of community medicine. We must remember that ancient China had no public health tradition — their stress had been on individual physical fitness and well-being.

Thus, the new emphasis on epidemiology and public health reaches beyond the rather narrow boundaries of individual physician-patient relationships as well as hospital-oriented missionary medicine. Such a new system of health care delivery presupposes the existence of a highly structured and de-centralized medical network linking rural villages with major urban centers. Moreover, it involves a clear chain of command and responsibility together with a team approach, integrating the various workers in the health field. Highly trained Western specialists with their technological capabilities work together with traditional physicians who have acquired a certain degree of modern medical knowledge. Furthermore, there are a host of paramedical workers involving nurses, mid-wives and medical corpsmen with varying degrees of training.

After reviewing the available reports, there is no doubt in my mind that the health care delivery system being used today in the People's Republic of China could serve as a useful model for the developing countries in Africa, Asia and Latin America. China's clear intention of giving top priority to the actual availability of medical and preventive care for its entire population ought to be carefully observed and assessed. The use of various paramedical personnel endowed with upward mobility rather than locked into a rigid system, should be studied in terms of the quality of care they are able to render and the supervision they require. Moreover, their medical education must be evaluated in relation to the new emphasis on practical matters instead of theoretical considerations.

Are there lessons in the Chinese model of health delivery which could apply to the United States? I believe there definitely are even though our societies are markedly different in their political, social and technological aspects. The People's Republic offers a large laboratory in which the modern tenets of community medicine can be studied and tested. Our rural areas and inner city ghettos could greatly benefit from a decentralized system of medical care delivered in part by paramedical people recruited from these areas. Their social awareness as well as their identification with the problems prevailing in the so-called "medically deprived" places would make them more effective patient's advocates and resourceful helpers. Training such people will require more flexibility in present academic admission policies, curriculum design and degree granting powers in order to allow for the already mentioned upward rise in the medical hierarchy. More important, however, would be the establishment of a proper framework in which each member of the health team could function with confidence and have the possibility of referral and consultation with another clearly identifiable level of more specialized care. The present sense of isolation experienced by many American practitioners, the rather haphazard relationship between generalists and specialists could benefit from a more structured system in which health care could be delivered more broadly without compromising quality.

The lack of proper statistics on the real impact of the new Chinese community medicine leaves us for the moment merely with superficial impressions about its true success and value. Furthermore, the great disruptions caused by the Cultural Revolution of the late 1960's are just now being mended and there is still a considerable degree of flux in the various social roles.

However, the soft nature of our present knowledge concerning Chinese medicine should not be a deterrent for new and more sustained efforts towards a better understanding of the health field in China. Without taking everything at face value, we should study the lessons already apparent in what I personally consider to be the most monumental effort in medical care ever launched in the history of mankind.

REFERENCES

Balme, Harold: *China and Modern Medicine,* a study in medical missionary development, London, London Missionary Society, 1921.

Cheng, T. H.: "Schistosomiasis in mainland China. A review of research and control programs since 1949," *Amer. J. Trop. Med. Hyg.* 20 (1971), 26-53.

Deutschle, K. W. and Eberson, F.: "Community medicine comes of age," *J. Med. Educ.* 43 (1968), 1229-1237.

Dimond, E. G.: "Medical education and care in People's Republic of China," *J.A.M.A.* 218 (1971), 1552-1557.

King, Maurice, ed.: *Medical Care in Developing Countries,* Nairobi and London, Oxford University Press, 1966.

Needham, J. and Lu, Gwei-djen: "Hygiene and preventive medicine in ancient China," *J. Hist. Med.* 17 (1962), 429-471.

Sidel, V. W.: "The barefoot doctors of the People's Republic of China," *New Engl. J. Med.* 286 (1972), 1292-1300.

Worth, R. M.: "Health in rural China: from village to commune," *Am. J. Hygiene* 77 (1963), 228-239.

Worth, R. M.: "Institution-building in the People's Republic of China: the rural health center," *East-West Center Review* 1 (1965), 19-34.

Some of the latest sources available in English translation can be found in the *Selections from China Mainland Press* (S.C.M.P.) published by the American Consulate General in Hong Kong and distributed by National Technical Information Service, U.S. Department of Commerce, Springfield, Va. 22151. They are:

"Peking medical team works in Jenan," from Sian, No. 28, 1971, *SCMP* 71-49 (December 1971), 145-146.

"Party Committee and Revolutionary Committee of Chishan Hsien, Shansi Province, perseveringly wage mass patriotic public health campaigns," from Peking Kuang-ming Jih-pao, March 24, 1972 *SCMP* 72-14 (April 1972), 112-114.

"Northwest China province of Chinghai makes progress in medical work," in Sining, April 8, 1972, *SCMP* 72-16 (April 1972), 165-166.

Chapter 11

(MEDICINE AND CHINESE SOCIETY)

Kenneth Levin

During a visit to China in the summer of 1971 I was profoundly affected, as indeed all my colleagues were, by the tremendous experiment in social engineering which has transformed that vast country and people from utter devastation into a progressive and flourishing society in just two decades. Yet the sheer magnitude of the achievement only began to dawn on me some months later during a brief visit to India, a country where, despite an agricultural "green revolution" which has more than doubled the amount of food since 1965, the starving and sick still lie dying in the streets, and where the long-term prospects are not very bright since the social causes of poverty, inequality, and suffering have only been muted by the increased crops, not eliminated.

During that visit to India one of my first impressions of China came back to me in sharp focus — the remarkable health and physical well-being of the people! Of the thousands of bright-eyed, curious children who thronged about us everywhere in China I could not remember one sign of hunger, or disease, or malnutrition anywhere — even in the remotest rural areas or the back alleyways of large cities. China has no more beggars, no more hungry and desperate people, and in addition is providing for the common health and well-being of everyone.

To those of us who live in advanced Western countries these achievements are too often taken much too lightly. They must be seen in terms of what China was like only a few years ago and in terms of what other developing countries are accomplishing. By way of contrast, W. H. Scott, a Canadian who had lived in China in the years before 1949, recalled how the children of Shanghai looked then:

The children . . . scurvy-headed children. Children with inflamed
red eyes. Children with bleeding gums. Children with distended
stomachs and spindly arms and legs . . . Children who had been
purposely deformed by beggars . . . children covered with horrible
sores upon which flies feasted . . . children having a bowel movement which, after much strain, would only eject tapeworms.[1]

This is certainly a far cry from the happy, healthy, industrious
children of Shanghai in 1972. How the changes have come about
is an important story. And how much they have meant in terms
of the basic human dignity and spiritual rebirth of one quarter
of the world's people is difficult to convey to those who have not
experienced it at first hand. Yet it seems to me that the healthy
condition of the Chinese people — seen through the programs,
achievements, and underlying philosophy of medical and health
care — would provide an interesting study of Chinese society in
microcosm. Health and medical care, along with virtually everything else, started at a very low level in 1949. The way the
programs have been organized, their successes and failures, the
philosophy of participation, all form a mirror of Chinese society
today — a society which gives top priority to widespread if
gradual improvement in the standard of living at the expense of
rapid growth in a few selected areas, and a society based on
self-reliance and self-sufficiency through hard work and the participation of all its members. Thus, while the use of acupuncture
as an anesthetic has received worldwide coverage, and while
attention of foreigners has been focused on pioneering work by
Chinese specialists in rejoining severed limbs, unprecedented
success in treatment of severe burns, and the world's first synthesis of biologically active bovine insulin by young Chinese
medical researchers, the Chinese are more concerned about and
prouder of their achievements in delivering a basic level of medical and health care to 750,000,000 poor people who twenty-three
years ago had virtually none. How they succeeded in this and
some of the far-reaching implications are subjects of this paper.

Priorities

In 1949 China lay in ruins, devastated by more than a
century of wars, invasions, internal corruption and colonial ex-

ploitation. These had in turn fostered widespread famines, epidemic diseases, and every kind of social humiliation and vice. One example was the terrible famine which engulfed Honan Province in 1943. The following is part of journalist Theodore White's eyewitness account:

> There were corpses on the road. . . . People chipped at bark, pounded it by the roadside for food; vendors sold leaves at a dollar a bundle. A dog digging at a mound was exposing a human body. Ghostlike men were skimming the stagnant pools to eat the green slime of the waters. . . . Refugees on the road had been seen madly cramming soil into their mouths to fill their bellies, and the missionary hospitals were stuffed with people suffering from terrible intestinal obstructions due to the filth they were eating.[2]

The Honan famine took between two and three million lives. Such disasters were part and parcel of life in traditional China — and still are in many parts of the world today. In the 1930's and 1940's over half of the people in China died before they reached the age of twenty-eight, and untold millions perished in infancy through ignorance and widespread superstition.[3] According to a report by Dr. William Y. Chen, an official of the United States Public Health Service, during the 1940's 4,000,000 people were dying of infections and parasitic diseases every year, while some 60,000,000 people were in need of medical care they could not obtain. Dr. Chen calculated that a minimum standard of one doctor for every 1,500 people and five hospital beds for every 1,000 persons would require 466,000 doctors and 3,500,000 beds,[4] while according to a report by the Chinese Medical Association China had, in the mid-1940's, only about 12,000 doctors (of whom only about 7,500 had formally completed a Western-type course), only 71,000 hospital beds, and facilities for turning out only 500 medical graduates per year. Furthermore, of the 12,000 doctors fully three-fourths were located in the main ports of the major coastal provinces where they made good livings off well-to-do patients.[5]

Obviously such staggering medical and health problems required drastic action by the new People's Government after 1949. The first steps were taken during the First National Health

Congress held in August of 1950. The Congress established several basic health principles which have formed the foundation of medical and health work ever since.

The first guideline was that health work must be directed primarily at the vast masses of poor working people, most of whom had never seen a doctor and were unaware of basic sanitation and health measures.

The second guideline was to give top priority to preventive medicine and the most basic medical and health services. Doctors and public health officials concentrated on eliminating diseases which strike in epidemic proportions by teaching basic hygienic principles, purification of water, treatment of human excrement before using it as fertilizer, and by giving vaccinations and inoculations against major diseases. The idea was to educate large numbers of the populace through rational explanations in order to achieve the maximum amount of cooperation.

In a June 1, 1972 interview with the New China News Agency, Professor Chu Fu-tang, 73, one of China's best-known pediatricians, recalled the early efforts in Peking to carry out this program.

> Shortly after the liberation of Peking, the people's government mobilized and organized the people for large-scale health and sanitation work. Refuse accumulated for over four or five hundred years from the Ming and Ch'ing Dynasties was finally cleared away. The sewage system was renovated and improved. Knowledge of environmental hygiene was taught far and wide.

These basic programs were surprisingly successful. The incidence of infectious skin diseases dropped drastically in just a few years through simple sanitation techniques. By 1957 virtually everyone was immunized against tuberculosis (by BCG), smallpox, diphtheria, pertussis, tetanus, plague, polio, measles, meningococcal meningitis, and encephalitis, while malaria and cholera occur only rarely if ever anymore. Today cancer and heart disease are the major causes of death in China — just as in advanced Western countries. And as far as general cleanliness and sanitation are concerned, no recent visitor to China has returned without remarking on how fanatically conscious the people are about cleanliness and sanitation.

Traditional Versus Modern Medicine

A third general guideline was to take advantage of the rich indigenous medical tradition by combining Chinese with Western medicine and by co-operating with the several hundred-thousand traditional Chinese herbalists and acupuncturists. Undoubtedly, part of the reason for this policy was absolute necessity. Without the traditional doctors most Chinese would have had no medical care at all. Besides, traditional medicine was a goldmine of centuries of knowledge and had given the world such drugs as ephedrine and the chaulmoogra nut which arrests leprosy. But Chinese traditional medicine was based on a profoundly different philosophical footing than modern science and was a highly individualistic art. Professional jealousy and competition resulted in little sharing of empirical knowledge gained by its practitioners — who saved it to pass on to a few selected apprentices, or to keep within the family. Moreover, traditional practice scarcely touched on basic anatomy or physiology and had only the barest knowledge of bacteriology, endocrinology, or parasitology (to name only a few), and was powerless to combat epidemic diseases. So, understandably there was a good deal of opposition and tension from the modern medical community.[6]

Nevertheless, by the mid-1950's the government made a full-scale commitment to the wholesale acceptance and study of traditional Chinese medicine, and began requiring modern doctors to study a certain amount of traditional theory and practice at the same time that traditional doctors were being taught the rudiments of modern Western medicine. Centers were also established for research into traditional medicine and techniques.

The resulting combination has led to some fascinating discoveries (of which acupuncture anesthesia is only one), and has made Chinese medical practice today rather unique in the world. A few examples: when we visited the East Wind Hospital (which emphasizes Chinese traditional medicine) in Soochow we were shown through a ward where bone fractures are treated by a combination of traditional and modern techniques. X-rays are used to determine the extent of damage and the procedure for reduction of the fracture. Then a system of Chinese splints is used rather than the heavy plaster casts found in the West, which often immobilize not only the area of the fracture but also the points above and below the break. The Chinese feel that through exercise of the nearby joints stiffness and muscle wastage are greatly reduced without endangering the knitting process of the fracture and that overall rehabilitation is speeded.

A second example is illustrated in a June, 1972 report by the New China News Agency, according to which the pediatrics department of the Peking Friendship Hospital has been achieving good results in treating bronchopneumonia in children by combining traditional Chinese and Western medicine. Since the disease is caused by bacterial and virus infection during a period of low physical resistance the doctors use herbal medicines, traditional methods of massage along the spinal column to increase the digestive function, and acupuncture and injections into needling points to increase the patient's appetite, to raise nutrition and therefore body resistance. Antibiotics are also used to combat inflammation of the lungs. According to the report all this has brought major improvements over the simple administration of antibiotics since the latter method does not take into account the problems of poor functioning of the cardiovascular system, spasms of the bronchioli, and the fact that asthma often continues. The traditional medications do have effects on these symptoms.

The tremendous and continuing popularity of traditional medicine was convincingly demonstrated to us on our visit to the East Wind Hospital in Soochow, where the outpatient clinic was jammed with people waiting for traditional prescriptions and treatments. There can be little doubt that the use of traditional medicine has greatly increased the availability and the quality of medical care in China today. Research is continuing to find new uses for acupuncture and to catalogue the various herbal medicines and what they really do. The West will undoubtedly benefit from the results of this research also in the near future.

The 'Mass Line'

A fourth general guideline which grew out of China's woeful inadequacies in medical facilities and trained personnel was that wherever possible medical workers should obtain the help of the whole population in carrying out medical and health programs. The first projects were mass campaigns to clean up the cities and to eliminate the so-called "four pests" (flies, rats, bedbugs, and mosquitoes — and in some areas lice and grain-eating sparrows). These campaigns received a lot of attention outside of China and were colorfully described to conjure up images of millions of people running around fanatically attacking rats with shovels or flies with rolled-up newspapers. How true these images were is difficult to judge.

From these rather crude beginnings the principle of enlisting everyone's co-operation and participation developed into a sophisticated concept known as the "mass line" in medical and health work. Basically the mass line means enlisting the help and obtaining the co-operation of everyone in the society to solve medical and health problems of all types. In other words, everyone has become a health worker. It also presupposes a tremendous educational effort because the masses must be made aware of the nature of the problems and what they can do to solve them. It is based on the teaching of Chairman Mao Tse-tung that when correct ideas are thoroughly understood by the masses of people they become tremendous forces for material change.

The concept seems simple and logical enough but putting it into practice was not easy at all. Many important people in the medical profession felt that using poorly trained personnel to carry out specialized health and medical responsibilities would lead to a tremendous variation in standards, and that spreading out the limited number of trained doctors throughout the country to teach basic medical and health programs would water down medical education and in the long run lower the quality of medical care. Little did anyone know just how successful the new philosophy would prove to be.

The earliest manifestations of the mass line were, as already mentioned, the mass health campaigns for personal and community hygiene, widespread innoculations and vaccinations, and the eradication of pests. But perhaps the most spectacular accomplishment of the use of the mass line to date has been the virtually complete elimination of venereal disease — which makes China (the most populous country and one of the poorest) the first major country in the world to do so.[7]

In order to attack venereal disease a transformation had to be brought about in the social and political factors causing it, the people had to be made aware of how to combat it, and the proper medicines and treatment techniques had to be made available. Venereal disease was introduced into China by the Portugese in the sixteenth century and rapidly spread throughout the country, mainly through colonialism, wars, and ravaging armies. Widespread poverty contributed to its growth as famines and desperation swelled the ranks of prostitutes and slave girls. So did other social evils such as the widespread use of opium and the common general low status of women with polygamy, concubinage and child-marriages.

After 1949 these social evils were eliminated. Colonialism was ended and likewise wars and invasions. The brothels were all closed down and prostitutes, drug addicts and other degenerate groups received treatment and rehabilitation courses in special centers.[8] The land was redistributed, people began to find work, while extreme poverty and the desperate behavior into which it leads people was gradually eliminated, so that the economic roots of prostitution and crime were swept away. At the same time the status of women was completely reversed with the passage of equal rights legislation and the new Marriage Law of 1950.[9] During this time penicillin was being produced around the clock.

These changes combined to greatly reduce the incidence of venereal disease, but the final attack came with the mobilization of thousands of medical and non-medical workers to carry out the mass line. A pilot experiment was set up in 1958 under the guidance of the Institute of Dermatology and Venereology and Dr. George Hatem, an American physician living in China, in Ningtu County, Kiangsi Province.[10] Briefly the project involved training cadres to educate the people of the area in the task of fighting venereal disease and breaking down resistance to treatment or to reporting symptoms. This was accomplished by appeals to patriotism, to the awful conditions of the past, and to pride in building a new society. Cadres' lectures usually took the following form:

> Syphilis is a legacy of the old society. Our party and people threw out the old ruling classes and their system that were the cause of our suffering. Our People's Government, our own government, wants to help us rid ourselves of the disease. It is no fault of your own that you are afflicted and no shame should be attached to it. Cure is sure and free. If you have any of the clues come for an examination. Comrades, we cannot take syphilis with us into socialism.[11]

Then simple questionnaires were distributed and explained in all the villages, communes, organizations and towns. These questionnaires asked ten questions about symptoms, an affirmative answer to any of which might indicate that the person had venereal disease. The emphasis was on getting everyone to report, by pointing out that neighbors and friends were doing so and by making a contest out of which localities would be the first to be rid of venereal disease. Then thousands of medical and health workers, cadres, Red Cross volunteers (of whom China has at least 2,000,000), students, and others were given a seven-day course in the principles of diagnosis and treatment. These trainees then waged a two-month campaign of discovery and treatment, under competent supervision wherever possible but for the most part on their own. The results convinced even the skeptics. A follow-up examination of Ningtu County by the Institute of Dermatology and Venereology showed that with only seven days of formal training, the volunteers had discovered and treated about 90 percent of the venereal disease cases in the area. The pilot project then served as the basis for similar programs nationwide and as a result venereal disease has been virtually eliminated from most areas and is under control throughout China.

In 1957 similar mass campaigns were organized for treatment of the six most common skin diseases (kala-azar, schistosomiasis, filariasis, hookworm, ringworm, and leprosy). Today, schistosomiasis and leprosy are the only ones left but even these are greatly reduced, and China will likely be the first country in the world to bring schistosomiasis under control.[12] Many other campaigns using the mass line were also undertaken, but one ongoing campaign is of especial interest, namely the task of birth control and family planning in the world's most populous nation.

With peace and prosperity after 1949 China underwent a veritable population explosion which rapidly threatened to wipe out all the gains made by the revolution. So the mass line was called into service in all its familiar forms. Education plays the primary role and the people are, as in all cases, given rational explanations for curtailing family size and practicing birth control. Many of the old values about the role of the family and about the bearing of many sons have had to be re-evaluated. In addition the educators point out that China simply has too many people, that too many children will wipe out the gains already made and will themselves suffer in the future, and that too many children are a burden on the parents and interfere with productive work.

Very little is known in the West about the population program in China, except that couples are "ordered" to marry late and have only two children. We found that there are no "orders," only that people are "encouraged" to wait until their mid-twenties. In fact we found that the average marriage age in many rural areas has now come up all the way to twenty-one! — which is still better than it used to be when teen-age marriages were common. Similarly there seem to be no economic sanctions on families with more than three children (as has often been reported) beyond what would exist if any family had more mouths to feed. Yet when we asked young people how many children they intended to have, the answer was always "two."

The Chinese point out that education and social awareness of the population problem are the primary reasons the problem is being brought under control. Oral contraceptives have been developed, however, and are widespread, both in pill form and in clever perforated sheets of rice paper from which they are detached one at a time like postage stamps and eaten. Intrauterine devices copied on Japanese models have been in use since about 1958. Vacuum-aspiration abortions are legal and available on demand, and we found that if an unmarried girl comes in for an abortion she is likely to receive special service consisting of a free lecture on morals. Mobile medical units in the countryside and paramedical personnel give lectures and lantern-slide shows, distribute contraceptives, perform IUD insertions, abortions, vasectomies and tubal ligations. Sterilization (both male and female) is available, but encouraged only for good reason and rationally explained.[13] Finally, female health workers in the cities and villages poll all the women of childbearing age in their neighborhood to find out what kinds of contraceptives they are using, and to help them plan families. The results of the mass program are really quite encouraging. Although the Chinese do not issue many statistics it has been estimated that the population growth rate has dropped from between 3 and 4 percent per year to about half that in the early 1970's, and continues to decrease. In cities, where education is easier, the growth rate seems to be almost zero, but in the countryside, where many traditional ideas and customs persist, the growth rate is still too high. Nevertheless, through the use of the mass line China should have the problem well under control in a few years.

Obviously, the key to the mass line is awakening people's awareness of the problems of the society and supplying them with the wherewithal and the incentive (or ethic) to help solve the problems. In China today most of that ethic is learned through reading the works of Mao Tse-tung. Mao's works exude confidence in the creative potential of the masses, call them to a great cause, preach selfless devotion to transforming China, and offer down-to-earth examples and anecdotes which peasants can understand, as well as methodological frameworks on which to base actions. An analysis of the thought of Mao Tse-tung is beyond the scope of this paper but a few examples from his writings may throw some light on the tremendous amount of co-operation and energy which go into bringing basic medical and health care to hundreds of millions of people. Everyone in China reads Mao's little essay entitled "Serve The People," in which he says: "We are wholly dedicated to the liberation of the people and work entirely in the people's interests. . . . And we need the vast majority of the people with us on the road to this objective."[14] Everyone also reads the essay on Norman Bethune, a Canadian surgeon who came to help the Chinese in their struggle against Japan, and died on the battlefield. In that essay Mao, obviously moved, says: "Comrade Bethune's spirit, his utter devotion to others without any thought of self, was shown in his great sense of responsibility in his work and his great warm-heartedness toward all comrades and the people. . . . We must all learn the spirit of absolute selflessness from him."[15] Dr. Bethune's spirit pervades medical and health work in China today, and "serving the people" is the main motivation for all actions. These values and exhortations to mass participation had to be taught at first, but now are an integral part of the makeup of Chinese life and work. Now everyone acts co-operatively because it works and all the people believe in it.

I have been trying to convey some feeling for what a Chinese means when he says that by studying the works of Mao Tse-tung he has been able to accomplish some concrete goal, because the reaction outside of China has often been one of mis-understanding and open derision. What the Chinese mean is that the values Mao teaches have raised their awareness of problems and their duty to the point that they know what to do about them. They call it "raising people's consciousness" or "putting politics in command." The closest phrase we have in English usage is probably "social awareness." It took politics or social awareness to do away with venereal disease. All the penicillin in the world would not have wiped it out if not preceded by awareness of the social and political causes of its existence and the co-operation of everyone to change these conditions.

The service ethic and the co-operative values also affect individual efforts in the medical field. In a recent talk at Wayne State University in Detroit, Dr. Joshua Horn recounted his ex-periences trying to describe to the members of the British Royal College of Surgeons how Chinese surgeons had been pioneers at rejoining severed limbs. "Why have the Chinese succeeded where we can't?" he was asked. "Is it better eyesight or manual dexterity or what?" His answer was that of course it had nothing to do with eyesight or dexterity. But to rejoin four severed fingers takes about seventeen hours of the most painstaking work, and then one of the veins may block and the surgeon will have to get out of bed and work for four more hours. The question really is what keeps him going? It is not money since doctors in China work on fixed salaries, and it is not fame since no one's name is ever mentioned apart from a team. The motivation of the doctor comes from his conviction that serving the people is the highest ideal of any person, and that in doing this work he is building China into a very good society. Dr. Horn then poked a little fun at his august audience by pointing out that the doctor got these values from his study of Mao Tse-tung's thought, so that the answer to the question "How can they do it where we have so far failed?" is really "By studying the works of Chairman Mao." "Of course," Dr. Horn concluded, "one could not have stated it thus in such hallowed surroundings."

Of course, the farthest-reaching implication of the mass line in medical and health work is that everyone in China has become a health-worker of sorts, and that if taken to its logical conclusion the mass line means the health community and part of the medical community should eventually become absorbed or completely immersed in the society at large. The practice of medicine and public health would thus become the responsibility of the community and one of those integral but invisible parts of the life style of every citizen. Of course, that is an ideal, but China has made a good beginning. And it has great implications for the nature of the medical and health work of the future.

Most people there already believe it is their responsibility to see that the health and well-being of their neighbors and friends are maintained. Even the foreign visitor can feel a certain calm security and serenity which this ethic has brought (the Chinese do *not* scurry around fanatically like hordes of blue ants); a sense that no one will harm you, or cheat you, or mistreat you, or steal from you; a sense that if you are in trouble, if you are sick, if you need help, someone will be there to help you. It is really a good feeling and one of the positive achievements of Chinese society. And the Chinese people really appreciate it.

The Training Of Medical And Health Personnel

Medical and health care are, however, not based on co-operative effort alone. Also necessary are skills, techniques, and practical knowledge which make possible the implementation of specific programs. So, while they have "put politics in command," the Chinese have also given top priority to training medical and health personnel. And in some of their programs they have embarked upon a truly revolutionary course which deserves serious consideration and careful appraisal.

Starting with only about 10,000 fully trained doctors in 1949, the Chinese immediately began to set up medical schools with departments of clinical medicine, public health, pharmacology, dentistry, and pediatrics. Courses were generally patterned after those of the United States and the Soviet Union and took from six to eight years to complete. According to one study, these medical schools had turned out about 150,000 fully trained medical doctors, 30,000 dentists, and 20,000 pharmacists by the time of the outbreak of the Cultural Revolution in 1966.[16] Up to about 1967, the same study estimates the training of approximately 500,000 secondary medical personnel — assistant doctors, pharmacists, nurses, midwives, etc. — with from two to four years of formal training.[17] In addition, during the Great Leap Forward period of 1958-1961 many doctors began to go into the countryside for periods of time to treat patients and to train peasants in basic medical and health work. Many local courses were set up to meet the needs of backward areas, and these turned out large numbers of medical and health workers of grossly varying degrees of competence. Counting these partly-trained people the grand total of all full-time medical and health workers in China by 1967 seems to have been in the neighborhood of 3,500,000, which amounts to about five full-time medical and health workers, many of very low competence for every 1,000 people in China.[18] The 1967 figures represent a large increase, but are certainly nothing sensational.

The government also built hundreds of new hospitals, most of them in cities or in county seats, but again the total number in relation to China's vast population has not been overly impressive. More basic was the program to establish a network of district health centers in the cities and similar county health centers in the countryside. The system, out of necessity, relied on local organizations and mass participation for success. Each street or neighborhood in a city and each village (or after communes were established in 1958 each production team) were to elect committees of residents to see that garbage and refuse were removed, that sidewalks and pavements were swept, and that general sanitation was maintained. These local committees helped organize the early pest-control and mass immunization campaigns. Each family was supposed to report all illnesses to its local unit, which then kept track of health problems and referred residents to nearby hospitals or clinics.[19] In the countryside the system was supposed to work the same way, with the health committees of production teams or brigades under supervision of the county health centers. But, for China's 600,000,000 rural peasants health and medical care were still very limited.

What had developed was a sort of three-tiered system of hospital and medical facilities. On the bottom level were the municipal clinics in the cities and the county health centers in the countryside, staffed for the most part by partially trained staff. On the middle level were the medium-sized hospitals in the cities and large towns. The rural equivalent was only a district health office staffed by research and public health officials. At the top were the few large medical centers and medical schools located in Peking and other major cities. Thus, despite a commitment to serve the masses, medical personnel tended to be educated in the cities and to remain near the best medical facilities which were located exclusively in the cities. As a result the system served best the people who lived in the cities — industrial workers, teachers, students, army people, and government workers — while the poor peasants who make up about 80 percent of China's population were still being largely neglected. These developments finally got to such an alarming point that in 1965 even Chairman Mao was moved to complain that the Ministry of Health had become a "Ministry of Health for Urban Overlords," and that in medical and health work the main emphasis must be put on the rural areas.

One of the important steps leading in this direction was the establishment in 1965 of mobile medical units, which consist of fully-trained physicians and assistants, nurses, technicians, sanitation and public health workers. In that year 160,000 city medical workers were formed into 10,000 mobile units to travel to certain parts of the countryside to provide care and treatment, but even more importantly to teach local people sanitation and public health, and to train paramedical personnel by the thousands. Today at any given time approximately one-third of the medical staffs of city hospitals and clinics are in the countryside. They usually remain on tour for about a year with brief vacations. The work is supposedly voluntary, but virtually everyone volunteers. Dr. Horn served on one of the first mobile units and has listed in his book the types of duties they performed: preventive and therapeutic health work, immunizations and vaccinations, teaching peasants how to protect cleanliness of water and to boil it before drinking, disposal and treatment of human and animal manures, ridding of lice, dispensing of medicine, training of local paramedical personnel, conducting of courses on planned parenthood, and finally, being "re-educated" by the whole experience — to understand peasant life and its needs so that health workers and peasants can best serve each other in the future.[20] Many Westerners would consider it a misuse of highly skilled people in having them perform rudimentary tasks in the countryside, but as they do these things the doctors are training thousands of local workers to do them in the future, and China is finally making good on its commitment to raise the level of medical care for all its people.

A second major step in the attempt to bring medical care to everyone in China right away has been the streamlining and shortening of medical training courses in the colleges. This step is relatively recent having been started in 1970. When we visited the Number Three Teaching Hospital attached to the Peking

University Medical School we found that the basic medical course has been cut from six years to about three, with graduates beginning clinical work after three years while continuing formal theoretical training on their own and in special night classes. In this regard formal medical education is in keeping with the rest of educational policy since the Cultural Revolution, namely to combine theory with practice and to serve the largest number of people possible.

The third major program for getting medical and health care to the masses has been the establishment on an unprecedented scale of new types of medical workers who are now known in rural areas as "barefoot doctors," in the cities as "red guard doctors," and in the factories as "worker doctors." Barefoot doctors receive crash courses in anatomy, first aid, public health work, innoculations, simple surgery, diagnosis, and the use of various kinds of Western and Chinese medicines. However, there is no limit or standard of knowledge for a barefoot doctor. Their learning process is continuous and their level of competence grows constantly. They are truly people's doctors, chosen from among the peasants, still working and being paid as if peasants, but handling basic medical and health work as it becomes necessary. Rural medicine has thus shifted from the county level to the commune, and more precisely to the brigade level. Each brigade determines its medical needs, chooses those from among its ranks whom it would like to have as doctors, and sees that they receive the proper training. The training is all done under the supervision of fully qualified physicians and public health officers and is subsidized by the government.

Having been entrusted with the responsibility of being *their* doctors by the local community and with the prevalence of the "serve the people" ethic the new paramedical personnel have taken up the important work with great fire and diligence, and have performed so competently that they have won the complete trust of the people who give them every bit of co-operation possible. As Horn is fond of pointing out the barefoot doctors are anything but poor quality doctors. They only do what their training has equipped them to do, but they do that so exceedingly well that within only a few short years everyone in China has been granted a basic level of medical care and has come to believe in the new system wholeheartedly. The goal is to have about two or three barefoot doctors for every rural production brigade. With the rate that these people are being trained the goal will be achieved within the next few years, for China is now producing more medical workers per year than any other country in the world.

The city counterparts of the barefoot doctor are of two types. Factory workshops choose members to receive the basic training, and when these "worker-doctors" return to the factory they continue to receive their worker's salary but spend part of their time treating the workers right on the job. Their "serve the people" attitudes are sometimes humorously impressive. We were always surprised, on our visits to factories, to see worker doctors snooping around, looking for sick people! Many treatments right in the workshop obviate the need for the worker to take time off to go to a clinic and thus help to reduce losses in production due to illness or injury. The same is true in the countryside where barefoot doctors are available for most common medical and health problems right in the fields.

The final category of the new type of medical worker is the "red guard doctor." These workers serve in city neighborhoods and operate "lane health stations." As already mentioned, each street, or lane, or neighborhood has an elected committee responsible for local services including health and sanitation work. Since the new program began, the committees have been recruiting retired residents, unemployed housewives, and part-time workers for training as red guard doctors to serve the local neighborhood. They work under the supervision of municipal clinics and perform the usual medical services.

The results of the barefoot doctor program have been a decentralization and widening of the scope of basic medical and health services, so that now virtually everyone in China is near a competent source of medical care. The movement is also fulfilling the tremendous task of providing care to such a huge population at a very low cost — a necessity for the success of any program in a poor peasant country.

The question of who does pay for the health and medical system is an interesting and revealing one. The government still pays the salaries of all full doctors and other highly-skilled medical and health workers. The barefoot doctors and their city counterparts, however, are paid by their local production unit as if they were still peasants or workers (in fact they are peasants and workers part of the time). They are not paid extra for their medical work but since they spend a large portion of their time doctoring and receive a regular farm or factory wage it amounts to having all the other local members contributing to their support in return for medical services. So communes in the country and factories in the city are footing the bill for a good deal of their medical care, but the cost of that care is incredibly low. On our visits to the countryside we noted that communes also save money by growing many of their own Chinese herbs and by producing simple medicines. Finally the patient also pays a share of his own medical costs, albeit a small one. Since 1968 a co-operative system has been established whereby each commune member pays a yearly fee (usually in the range of a dollar) to his local health facility, and then pays about two or three cents for each visit with medications not costing extra. This way the local medical units have become independent of state aid and the control which inevitably accompanies that. Thus the answer to the question of who pays is really (as always) that the people do, but they are paying for their very own medical system, one which is not only efficient but also one they can afford. One other related point about who pays is that everyone contributes in ways which are essential if the system is to work, by giving voluntary time to health and sanitation work, by being thrifty and not taking undue advantage of the system, and by the universal ethic of serving the people in all actions. Thus the system operates cheaply and efficiently because the people do not abuse it.

CONCLUSION

Even the most skeptical of recent visitors to China have been impressed with the kind of quiet competence which seems to prevail in medical and health care. From the cleanliness of the streets to the use of antibiotics along with acupuncture one has the feeling that the medical problem, if not solved completely, is rapidly getting there. One senses this in the healthy faces and the bright-eyed children. To deliver a basic level of medical and health care to one quarter of mankind, at low cost and at the time it is needed has been and continues to be a mammoth undertaking. Yet while there are still problems — a good deal of backwardness and a shortage of personnel and sophisticated equipment — the Chinese are on the verge of turning that task into a reality, not somewhere in the far-distant utopian future or on the theoretician's drawing board, but in the real world of Chinese life today. We in the United States ought to take note and learn what we can from the Chinese experience.

FOOTNOTES

[1]W. H. Scott, *Eastern Horizon Magazine,* Vol. V. No. 6. June 1966 quoted in Joshua S. Horn, M. D. *Away With All Pests: An English Surgeon in People's China, 1954-1969* (Monthly Review Press, New York, 1969), p. 19.

[2]Theodore White & Anallee Jacoby, *Thunder Out of China* (W. Sloane Associates, New York, 1961), pp. 169 & 171.

[3]"Ignorant gamps often attended at childbirth, and their practice of biting through the umbilical cord and applying cow-dung to the stump caused many babies to die of tetanus. . . ." Horn, *Away With All Pests,* p. 125.

[4]William Y. Chen, "Medicine and Public Health," *China Quarterly* No. 6 April-June 1961.

[5]Szeming Sze, *China's Health Problems* (Washington, D.C., Chinese Medical Association, 1943), p. 18.

[6]A report on that struggle is beyond the scope of this survey, but for an able discussion of the problems of combining the traditional and modern forms see: Ralph C. Croizier, "Traditional Medicine in Communist China: Science, Communism, and Cultural Nationalism," *The China Quarterly* (July-September 1965); reprinted also as a pamphlet by the *Far East Reporter,* New York City.

[7]Some medical experts estimate that as many as a million and a half cases of untreated syphilis are at large in the United States, while gonorrhea there is now the second most prevalent communicable disease, just behind—and gaining on—the common cold.

[8]An interesting description by Dr. George Hatem of this aspect of the campaign may be found in Edgar Snow, *Red China Today: The Other Side of the River* (Vintage Books, New York, 1971), pp. 271-272.

[9]Horn, *Away With All Pests,* pp. 83-93.

[10]The following is a brief summary of Hatem's detailed report of the results: "With Mao Tse-tung's Thought as the Compass for Action in the Control of Venereal Diseases in China," *China's Medicine* No. 1 (October 1966), pp. 52-68.

[11]Ibid., p. 61.

[12]Schistosomiasis is a debilitating disease caused by a liver fluke which enters humans through the skin and lodges in the liver and intestines. The eggs are passed in the feces, hatch into larvae on contact with water, and enter into snails where they mature before returning to human carriers to complete the cycle. According to the World Health Organization approximately 250,000,000 people throughout the tropical world suffer from the disease. For a description of the mass campaigns to rid China of schistosomiasis, see Horn, *Away With All Pests,* pp. 94-106.

[13]No billboards in China offer free transistor radios to those who will submit to sterilization—as I have seen in India.

[14]Mao Tse-tung, "Serve the People," *Selected Works of Mao Tse-tung,* English Edition, Vol. III (1965), pp. 227-228.

[15]Mao Tse-tung, "In Memory of Norman Bethune," *Selected Works of Mao Tse-tung,* English Edition, Vol. II (1965), pp. 337-338.

[16]Leo A. Orleans, "Medical Education and Manpower in Communist China." in C. T. Hu, ed. *Aspects of Chinese Education* (Teachers' College Press: Columbia University, New York, 1969), p. 30.

[17]*Ibid.,* pp. 36-37.

[18]*Ibid.,* pp. 39-40.

[19]Snow, *Red China Today: The Other Side of the River,* p. 304.

[20]Horn, *Away With All Pests,* pp. 130-146.

Chapter 12

BAREFOOT DOCTORS IN CHINA: PEOPLE, POLITICS, AND PARAMEDICINE

Paul G. Pickowicz

IT IS SIGNIFICANT, I THINK, that this conference on Chinese Medicine has been organized, and so many of those in the medical profession in the United States have expressed interest in the topic. Specifically, this paper deals with the most significant medical and health force in China — the barefoot doctor, and in doing so it takes account of the most significant medical book in China — *The Instruction Manual for Barefoot Doctors*. This conference comes at a time when direct contact between the Chinese and American people is once again underway after an interlude of more than two decades. The general absence of American visitors to China over the last twenty years has had the effect of dramatizing for recent American visitors the enormous changes which have taken place in China. European, Canadian, and Japanese travellers to China since 1949 were quite competent in reporting the astounding changes taking place in New China, but for a variety of reasons these accounts were largely ignored in America. Suddenly it is as though Americans have discovered China, and tales of Chinese miracle working have astounded American readers since the ping pong period began in the Spring of 1971. Americans seem to thrive on excesses. First, little reliable American news for twenty years, then a sudden deluge of untrained reporting which seems to have had the singular effect of making China the latest fad.

It is a happy coincidence, however, that one of the topics

which has received the most attention is the development of medical and health practice in People's China. A discussion of medical and health policies is an excellent place to begin an overall consideration of the significance of the Chinese revolution for both America and the Third World. The conflicts and trends in medicine and health are symbolic of similar phenomenon in literature and the arts, and even in the communist party itself.[1]

The full impact of health and medical delivery in China cannot be appreciated without comparisons and contrasts to other locations and other times. Recent reports from China have betrayed the journalists' lack of understanding of the health situation in China during the decades before 1949. In a land where peasants still account for 80 percent of the population, even the most rudimentary health care was completely unknown before the founding of the People's Republic. The English surgeon Joshua Horn, a longtime resident of China, has written:

> Poverty and ignorance were reflected in a complete lack of sanitation as a result of which water-borne diseases such as typhoid, cholera, dysentery, took a heavy toll. Worm infestation was practically universal, for untreated human and animal manure was the main and essential soil fertilizer. The people lived on the fringe of starvation and this so lowered their resistance to disease that epidemics carried off thousands every year. The average life expectancy in China in 1935 was stated to be about twenty-eight years. . . . There were no preventive inoculations against infectious diseases, and from time to time epidemics of smallpox, diphtheria, whooping cough and meningitis swept through the countryside with devastating results. Lice and poverty went hand in hand, and with them louse-borne diseases such as typhus fever.[2]

By 1949 the number of modern physicians was less than one per 100,000 people, but most of these doctors lived in the large cities. The general situation in the countryside was made more unbearable by the combination of warlordism, civil war, foreign invasion, and natural disaster. Recalling a three year famine which devastated Szechuan Province in southwest China from 1929 to 1932, Edgar Snow wrote, "There for the first time I saw children dying by the thousands, in a famine which eventually took more than five million lives but was scarcely noticed in the West."[3]

These ghastly recollections bring to mind events of recent years and months in India, Pakistan, and Bangladesh. When we discuss China in any context we should remember that twenty-five years ago there was little to distinguish social conditions in China from those in the South Asian subcontinent. A comparison of developments in both areas over the last twenty years is most enlightening. Finally, we should not refrain from making comparisons between China and the advanced industrial societies such as the United States. One of the fruits of America's "discovery" of China is a willingness to admit that we have much to learn from China. Dr. Paul Dudley White reported after his recent visit to China that in the delivery of health care the Chinese are in fact ahead of the United States. Our approach to China has undergone great changes. Our arrogance in dealing with the "Sick Man of Asia" has been tempered by humility these days. The Chinese people have the dignity and respect of a nation which has stood up and taken a firm grasp of its destiny. They take pride in the fact that the people have done it themselves.

It should not be surprising then, that the specific topic of this paper is one which is of interest to both Chinese and Americans. Barefoot doctors are neither "barefoot" nor "doctors"; they are really paramedical personnel. More and more Americans are beginning to discuss the question of paramedics in socio-political rather than medical terms. Why is it that in America, the richest and most advanced country in medical technology, there are millions who do not have adequate medical and health care because they cannot afford it, or because there are not enough medical personnel with proper credentials to treat them? Many ask whether it is necessary to spend years acquiring an M.D. degree to be qualified to treat common illnesses. Powerful lobbies have resisted any trend towards "lowering standards." A related problem is the tendency for medical students to gravitate towards specialized training where the money is, rather than towards general practice where the people are. Training more M.D.s does not seem to be the answer. It takes too long, and many have no interest in general practice. This essay is about China's approach to the same problem. In China after 1949 the problems were much more exaggerated. For the 500,000,000 peasants in the rural areas even the most basic health care was unknown, and there was no money to pay for medical care. There were a number of Western trained physicians, but they were confined to a few urban areas. In the countryside there were some traditional Chinese medical practitioners who specialized in herbal medicine and acupuncture, but they were, for the most part, servants of the landed gentry. Paramedical personnel, who came to be known as barefoot doctors, were a vital part of the solution to this almost hopeless problem. In this paper I will discuss the origin of Chinese paramedical programs in general, but focus on an evaluation of barefoot doctors since the origins of the Chinese Cultural Revolution in 1965. It was on June 26, 1965 that Mao Tse-tung wrote, "In medical and health work, put the stress on the rural areas." In this discussion I will draw upon my personal experience in China during June and July 1971, as well as a study of the important documents which have appeared in the Chinese press on the subject of barefoot doctors. Finally, I will discuss, for the first time in the West, the contents of *The Instruction Manual for Barefoot Doctors* (Ch'ih-chiao i-sheng p'ei-hsun-chiao-ts'ai) in order to determine the precise nature and scope of their work.[4]

Origins of Paramedical Work in China

Through the centuries necessity always dictated that China's peasants employ the services of paramedical personnel. In most every village there was some sort of medical consultant whose medical knowledge was a combination of practical experience and herbal formulas passed down through the family. Unhappily their practice was ridden with superstition and myth. Of the witch-doctors Dr. Horn wrote, ". . . their practise of biting through the umbilical cord and applying cow-dung to the stump caused many babies to die of tetanus. . . ."[5] In the late 1920s, however, when the Chinese communists were establishing rural base areas in south China, they were faced with the challenge of wiping away superstitions of all sorts, and providing fundamental health services for the millions of peasants living within the Soviet areas. In 1944 Mao Tse-tung wrote:

> Among the 1,500,000 people of the Shensi-Kansu-Ninghsia Border Region, there are more than 1,000,000 illiterates, there are 2,000 practitioners of witchcraft, and the broad masses are still under the influence of superstition . . . the human and animal mortality rates are both very high . . . in such circumstances, to rely solely on modern doctors is no solution. Of course modern doctors have advantages over doctors of the old type, but if they do not concern themselves with the sufferings of the people, do not unite with the thousand and more doctors and veterinarians of the old type in the Border Region and do not help them to make progress, then they will actually be helping the witch doctors. . . . There are two principles for the united front: the first is to unite, and the second is to criticize, educate, and transform.[6]

Even in those days the primary emphasis was on combining the positive elements of both Western and Chinese medicine, establishing preventive medicine and health education as a top priority, and encouraging modern doctors to train the peasants themselves in the kinds of basic medical practices which would have the most impact on the people. This type of program was embodied in the spirit of Dr. Norman Bethune, the famed Canadian physician who came to China in 1938 to serve in the communist Eighth Route Army during the war of resistance against Japan. During this period it was reported that often he volunteered transfusions from his own blood, designed makeshift medical equipment from whatever building material at hand, and trained whole clinics of peasant paramedics as he travelled about. His death in 1939 as a result of blood poisoning prompted the writing of one of Mao Tse-tung's most famous articles, "In Memory of Norman Bethune." He wrote, "Comrade Bethune's spirit, his utter devotion to others without any thought of self, was shown in his great sense of responsibility in his work and his great warmheartedness towards all comrades and the people. Every communist must learn from him. . . . No one who returned from the front failed to express admiration for Bethune whenever his name was mentioned, and none remained unmoved by his spirit."[7] My reading of the documents relevant to barefoot doctors since 1965 indicates that Bethune's name and spirit are as much a model for paramedics today as they were in 1939.

After the victory of the revolution in 1949 the communists were obviously in a position they had never before experienced. They controlled the whole country, enjoyed the popular support of the people, and were faced with the monumental task of organizing and reconstructing the nation. While the movement to train paramedical personnel in the rural areas did not come to a halt, there was a new drive to make functional the urban medical schools which were in the hands of communist administrators for the first time. Gradually there emerged debate and even tension between these two approaches: one called for integration of traditional Chinese and modern medicine, and the widespread training of peasants who would function as part time medical workers; the other called for centralizing medical development in the cities, and training medical specialists along Western lines. Of course neither approach precludes simultaneous development of the other; rather it has been a question of which approach takes precedence over the other. In periods of Maoist mass campaigns such as the Great Leap Forward of 1958-1959, the Socialist Education Movement of 1961-1962, and the Great Proletarian Cultural Revolution from 1965 to the present, the focus has been on the countryside and the training of peasant paramedics to handle the movement in preventive medicine and basic medical care. And during the entirety of the period from the late 1920s to the present the issue of health care delivery has always been raised and discussed foremost as a political question.

A Case Study: Communes Outside Shanghai

Perhaps the best method of defining barefoot doctors, describing their training, and suggesting the scope of their activities is to use as a case study the rural area outside Shanghai which I visited in June 1971. It was in this location that the term barefoot doctor was coined by local peasants during the Cultural Revolution. With such regional diversity, however, it is impossible to say that any example is typical for all China; rather, this case study is simply an indication of the direction in which the medical and health program is going.

Shanghai is not only a city, but also a national administrative unit which governs itself apart from the province in which it happens to be located. Peking has a similar sort of status. The Shanghai administrative region includes the metropolitan city of about six million people, and the surrounding countryside which contains almost four million peasants who live in the ten counties outside the city. In this rural area there are over 100 people's communes with an average population of between 25 and 30 thousand each. Hungchiao Commune where I visited has about 27,000 people, and Chiangchen Commune, about whose medical program so much has been written, has 28,000 people.[8] Each commune is broken down into a number of production brigades which are simply a collection of seven or eight villages. Hungchiao has 15 brigades, and Chiangchen has 21. Both communes have a total of more than 100 villages. The more than 100 communes outside Shanghai have a total of 2500 production brigades. The brigades are particularly important because it is there that most of the public services are provided for the people. One village is selected as brigade headquarters, and chances are it will contain an elementary school and a small health clinic.

Beginning in 1952 when the enormous people's communes were created there was a massive Maoist oriented health campaign initiated to train part time paramedical personnel from among the ranks of the peasantry. Over 10,000 professional medical people from Shanghai city were organized into mobile teams for the purpose of training rural paramedics. Many young people received ten months of training at a county medical school, but even more were trained by the mobile medical teams. When they returned to the various communes their task was to organize and lead mass health campaigns to purify water supplies, rid the area of insect pests, treat human and animal waste before it was used as fertilizer, and to inoculate the people against various diseases. They also had some skill in diagnosing and treating common illnesses, and using some of the traditional techniques of herbal medicine and acupuncture. In the delivery of health care they were to serve as the middle strata between the handful of full time experts at commune and county hospitals, and the folk doctors and midwives at the village level. These paramedical people were stationed at the brigade level, and by June 1960 there were 3900 paramedical people for the 2500 production brigades around Shanghai. Chiangchen Commune sent 19 people to be trained in paramedicine, and of these six were sent to the county medical school for a ten month course of study. Soon each brigade in Chiangchen Commune had its own health station. The enormity of this effort nationwide can only be appreciated when one learns that there are over 70,000 people's communes in China containing a total population of over 550 million peasants. There were problems for this program as well as for the Great Leap Forward as a whole. There were many who, for a variety of reasons, were opposed to the Great Leap in general, and when economic setbacks occurred in the late 1950s and 1960s the Great Leap was blamed. According to documents released during the Cultural Revolution the program to train part time paramedical people was among those scrapped by the opponents of the Great Leap. A report made in August 1961 ordered this new force in the countryside outside Shanghai to discontinue their medical work. The number of health workers of this sort was reduced from 3900 to just over 300. But another Maoist mass campaign called the Socialist Education Movement was launched from 1963 to 1964 and the number of health workers outside was raised from 300 to 2300.[9] A showdown was shaping up.

By 1965 it was clear that the question of the correct orientation of medical and health work in China would become one of the many important issues of the Cultural Revolution. The political questions of the health and medical program (which will be discussed later) were basically the same as the political questions of economic planning, government administration, party organization, and educational development. In each case Mao seemed to be saying that the first priority should be to serve the peasants and build up the rural areas. On June 26 he issued the well known directive, "In medical and health work, put the stress on the rural areas." Mobile medical teams were once again sent to the countryside around Shanghai to cooperate with county authorities for the purpose of training paramedical personnel. It was precisely in this context that the term "barefoot doctor" was first used. Although it is difficult to pinpoint the approximate date of its first use, the term first appeared in the national news media in September 1968. This article in *Hung Ch'i* (Red Flag), the main theoretical journal of the Chinese Communist Party, opened by introducing the term to readers throughout the country: "Barefoot doctors is an affectionate title that the poor and lower-middle peasants on the outskirts of Shanghai have given to health workers who spend part of their time farming, and part in medical work."[10] Beginning in the spring and summer of 1969 a flurry of articles elaborated on the subject of barefoot doctors. By the time the *Hung Ch'i* article was published in 1968 the number of barefoot doctors operating in the farmlands outside Shanghai had risen to 4500 — an average of 1.8 for each brigade. They, in turn, had trained over 29,000 health workers who are less skilled than the barefoot doctors and function at the village rather than the brigade level.

In Chiangchen Commune, for example, there were 28 barefoot doctors by September 1968, and by January 1970 there were 44 barefoot doctors, or two for each of the 21 brigades.[11] In Hungchiao Commune where I toured in June 1971 there were a total of more than 200 medical and health personnel, including a full-time, professional hospital staff at the commune level, about two barefoot doctors for each of the 15 brigades, and an average of nearly two health workers in each of the 108 villages. For Hungchiao then, the medical and health picture looks something like this: 1) a fairly sophisticated hospital at the commune level to serve the 27,000 people. The staff at the hospital is full time, and is capable of performing relatively minor operations such as appendectomies, and vasectomies. 2) About two barefoot doctors in each brigade who serve, on a part time basis, the approximately 1700 people who inhabit the seven villages of each brigade. 3) An average of nearly two health workers primarily responsible for general health and sanitation information, and preventive medicine campaigns in each village of approximately 250 people. Therefore at the brigade level in Hungchiao Commune there are nearly 14 health workers and two barefoot doctors for the 1700 people who inhabit the average brigade. It is probably fair to say that this type of program is the goal for all the communes outside Shanghai, and that most communes are already within reach. In fact the latest figures for the 2500 brigades surrounding Shanghai indicate that there are now a total of 6000 barefoot doctors.[12] This does not mean that the situation is equally as good in all parts of China. As China's largest city, Shanghai is in a good position to supply medical equipment and training to the outlying areas. The communes outside Shanghai are also relatively prosperous, and therefore have more resources to sink into medical and health programs. The real test of the Maoist medical campaign will be in the poorer and more remote areas of north, northwest, and southwest China. But at least the figures for the outlying areas of Shanghai give us some feeling for the direction in which the total national program is headed.

To better define barefoot doctors a number of specific questions should be asked:

WHERE DO THEY COME FROM? One of the primary methods of defining barefoot doctors is by their social origins. It is intended that they should be, for the most part, recruited from among the ranks of the peasantry, or as it was put in *Hung Ch'i*, ". . . the poor and lower-middle peasants understand that the power in medical and health work must be in their own hands."[13] It is generally believed in China that if worker and peasant culture is to be brought about it will not do to have medical or other important services provided to workers and peasants by experts and professionals who are themselves not of worker or peasant origin. It is also believed that medical and health campaigns are more effective when they are led by local people who are trusted by the village or brigade populace as a whole. The prospective barefoot doctors are selected by local people primarily on the basis of attitude and enthusiasm. Most candidates do seem to have a primary or junior high school education, although there are frequent reports of successful barefoot doctors who had only 2½ years of formal education before beginning medical and health training. Most of the barefoot doctors are young — the average age at Chiangchen Commune is 23 years, but there are reports of barefoot doctors as old as 64 years.[14] The records indicate that there are a large number of women barefoot doctors, but it is difficult to determine whether or not they constitute more or less than 50 percent.

WHAT IS THEIR STYLE OF WORK? The documents seem to indicate that no one can really be considered a barefoot doctor unless he or she is also engaged in agricultural work alongside fellow villagers. One report suggests, "On ordinary days, the barefoot doctors spend about half their time in farm work."[15] In practice I suspect that more than 50 percent of their time is spent in medical practice. This matter is viewed by the Chinese as a political question. There is no question that the Chinese find it difficult to respect any able bodied person who does not spend at least part of the time doing manual work. Teachers, intellectuals, scientists, artists, and government bureaucrats are encouraged to get out to the communes during the summer, or to volunteer for revolutionary sabbaticals which involve six month work and study periods in May Seventh Cadre Schools. While it is true that the Chinese are suspicious of urban experts, they are also concerned that worker or peasant children who receive training and become experts in the cities will also develop a negative attitude towards manual work, and thereby abandon their class. It is now expected that young peasants who go to the city to receive specialized training will come back to the villages to serve the local people rather than remain in the city to seek reputation and career. The Chinese seem to define "class" more on the basis of how one thinks and acts rather than on the basis of one's concrete class background. Therefore, it is possible for a peasant's son to work against the interests of the peasantry, and conversely for an intellectual's daughter to "become" a peasant by acting like a peasant, and serving the peasant community. This necessitates working in the fields no matter what one does. This whole question may seem irrelevant to Western medical experts, but it must be kept in mind the damage done by careerism in a society like India where many skilled young people first become medical specialists of one sort or another, and then seek out the best paying urban locations in India and even foreign countries such as England.

How ARE THEY PAID? The salary of barefoot doctors varies from commune to commune and from brigade to brigade. The general guideline is as follows: ". . . income is kept on a level with that of peasants having similar labor power."[16] In Tungping Brigade of Chiangchen Commune barefoot doctors made 300 yuan in 1967 ($120.). Of this total 100 yuan were earned as a result of work done in the fields, and 200 yuan were paid by the brigade as a subsidy. But since barefoot doctors in this brigade collected about 125 yuan in home calls (injections, child deliveries, etc.), the brigade actually paid out only 75 yuan. In another brigade, Minli, production was not so high in 1967 and the barefoot doctors made only about 200 yuan (54 yuan from agricultural work, 92 yuan from home calls, and 61 yuan in brigade subsidy).[17] The cost to the peasant community for these services is minimal. The total population of the two brigades is 2600. The subsidies and home calls for the two locations amount to 353 yuan, or an average of .13 yuan per peasant; the subsidies alone come to only 136 yuan or an average of .05 yuan per peasant. The reason that incomes vary from brigade to brigade and year to year is simply due to differences in total agricultural production. The method of payment in the commune system is to divide the surplus among the peasants on the basis of the amount of work done. Barefoot doctors seem to be paid in accordance with what they would have made had they been doing agricultural work all year. While this system insures that the barefoot doctors will earn no more than the average peasant, it may discriminate against women barefoot doctors. Ablebodied male peasants are awarded the maximum of ten work points, while ablebodied women are consistently awarded less. It may be then, that women barefoot doctors receive a smaller subsidy than men barefoot doctors even though they do the same work. I have seen no comparative figures for men and women barefoot doctors, however, and would be hesitant to conclude that this inequality exists in fact.

WHERE, FOR HOW LONG, AND BY WHOM ARE THEY TRAINED? Barefoot doctors seem to be trained in a number of places. Some are trained locally at the commune hospital by either modern physicians who have come from the city to serve for a period of years in the commune hospital, or by mobile teams of medical experts who have come from Shanghai and travel from county to county for the explicit purpose of training barefoot doctors. Other potential barefoot doctors leave the commune to study at county hospitals and medical schools, or even municipal hospitals in Shanghai. During the Cultural Revolution it was common to see mobile medical teams organized and led by the People's Liberation Army, which is quite active in medical work throughout the country. The amount of training received by beginning barefoot doctors also seems to vary. For those who study locally, the beginning orientation course seems to last about two months. The more I studied the question, however, the clearer it became that the formal classroom training of barefoot doctors was an ongoing process. One's ability to practice medicine depends on the amount of training received. The point is that the Chinese regard as mistaken any method of training medical personnel which confines them to the classroom for years at a time. Even after the most basic course, the barefoot doctors are skilled enough to carry on *some sort* of medical and health work. In fact, medical and health leaders in China argue that experience gained through actual practice is as important as classroom training. When barefoot doctors come back from two or three months of coursework they continue to learn from those in their local area who have more experience, and much of this training is informal. Many who received basic training during the Great Leap Forward in 1958 were qualified to attend more advanced courses during the Cultural Revolution of the mid-1960s. A fairly typical case is that of a barefoot doctor at Chiangchen Commune:

> He was an activist in the public health campaign to eliminate pests and prevent diseases during the Great Leap Forward in 1958. He was sent by the commune to study for ten months at a county

medical school. He then worked in the commune clinic for several years, and later attended a seven month course in surgery. Today he is able to do herniorrhaphy, sterilization and other operations even with simple medical apparatus.[18]

Eventually this process of training leads to the selection of a few skilled barefoot doctors to attend more sophisticated and advanced medical programs in the city. Once again the case of Chiangchen Commune is illustrative of this process. In 1968, for example, when there were 28 barefoot doctors, the commune selected an additional 144 health assistants at the village level (approximately one per team). All of these health assistants continued to work in the fields part time. The barefoot doctors are the ones primarily responsible for training the health assistants in preventive medicine, and from among the 144 sixteen advanced to the status of barefoot doctors, bringing the total of barefoot doctors to 44. The barefoot doctors work in the countryside for at least two to three years before any are selected to attend more advanced urban medical programs which are often two to three years in length. After completing a 2-3 year medical program in the city, the students return to the communes to spend what amounts to full time on advanced medical work, and it appears that they lose their status as barefoot doctors. They are no longer paramedical personnel, but rather, experts trained from among the ranks of the peasantry.

WHAT IS THE CONTENT OF THE TRAINING COURSES? Of course the content varies in accordance with the previous training of the barefoot doctor, but a rough outline can be given here. A more complete discussion of the capabilities of the barefoot doctors is contained in the final section of this essay which deals with the *Instruction Manual for Barefoot Doctors*. Suffice it to say that the training falls into four broad categories: prevention, diagnosis, treatment, and nursing. A beginning barefoot doctor is likely to concentrate on prevention. A course of this sort might discuss basic human anatomy, purification of water supplies, treatment of human and animal waste used as fertilizer, and pest control. The diagnosis, treatment and nursing instruction comes in more advanced courses. But in all training the emphasis is placed on common problems in the local areas rather than on relatively rare medical problems, or problems peculiar to a distant part of the nation. There is also an ongoing attempt to combine the techniques of modern medicine with those of traditional Chinese medicine. For the Chinese this is a political question. They are extremely critical of those who are slavish to foreign medical developments, and very proud of traditional practice in herbal medicine and acupuncture which they are convinced have great use. China is one of the few Third World countries which has refused to throw out the tenets of traditional medicine in favor of all out Westernization, and their health and medical service is richer for it .The average barefoot doctor in Chiangchen Commune has been described in the following way:

> After more than two years of practice, they have made remarkable progress in their medical skill. All of them can prescribe around 100 medicinal preparations, and diagnose and cure around 100 common ailments of frequent occurrence in the rural districts. They can perform acupuncture on more than 100 points on the human body. They can cure such common but serious illnesses in the rural districts as measles, pneumonia, and pleurisy. Some of them have shown more in practical work than some of the doctors in the commune clinic, who are graduates of medical schools but lack practical medical experience.[19]

In Shenmu County, Shensi Province in the northwestern part of China a medical school for barefoot doctors offers a two year program. During the two year period the students spend three months each year doing agricultural work in their villages, three months each year doing agricultural work at the medical school, and six months each year in the classroom. The hospital administrators have reported that the income from the agricultural work was sufficient to cover the costs of administration, laboratory tests, tuition, living expenses and the cook's wages. In a country as poor as China it is rather important that medical and health ventures of this sort be as self-sufficient as possible. In the 1967-68 period the school turned out 58 barefoot doctors.[20]

WHAT IS THE ROLE OF PROFESSIONALS? While it is true that the Chinese appear to be suspicious of urban specialists in general, it is also true that they must depend on these highly skilled people for many things. All the available evidence seems to indicate that the barefoot doctors are, at every level, trained by medical professionals. Ever since the 1930s Mao Tse-tung has viewed experts and technocrats in two ways. On the one hand professionals tend to become elitist. In the medical field this simply means that highly skilled professionals seek to increase their specialization, enhance their reputations and careers, and cling to the cities rather than serve the rural people whose health and medical needs are basic yet crucial. On the other hand, Mao has expressed his faith in the ability of intellectuals and professionals to reorient themselves ideologically and serve in the best interests of the people as a whole rather than pursue career interests. As mentioned before, the voluntarist strain in Maoist thinking also recognizes the possibility that peasants who acquire specialized training in the cities might also betray the interests of their class.

The reports from Chiangchen Commune give credit to an urban medical professional who was able to avoid careerism and elitism:

> In Chiangchen Commune the medical training of 28 barefoot doctors was undertaken by a doctor at the commune clinic who had come from a city medical school. In the last few years he has established warm class bonds with the poor and lower-middle peasants. He understood that in carrying out Chairman Mao's brilliant instruction, "In medical and health work, put the stress on the rural areas," he should not only act as a rural doctor himself but regard the training of barefoot doctors as an important task. He wrote a large amount of simplified teaching materials for medical work and public health in the villages, recommended some popular medical works suitable for villages, organized the barefoot doctors to help each other, and in particular gave them guidance on how to study on their own so that they could quickly cross the threshold through practice. In fact it is not difficult to cross the threshold.[21]

Mao Tse-tung himself was so impressed when he read the details of this report that he wrote:

> From the example of this doctor who came to the village from the city it can be seen that the majority or the vast majority of the students trained in the old schools and colleges can integrate them-

selves with the workers, peasants and soldiers, and some have made inventions or innovations; they must, however, be reeducated by the workers, peasants, and soldiers under the guidance of the correct line and thoroughly change their old ideology. Such intellectuals will be welcomed by the workers, peasants, and soldiers. If you doubt this, think of that doctor in Chiangchen Commune, Chuansha County, Shanghai.[22]

HOW MANY CASES DO BAREFOOT DOCTORS TREAT? In Chiangchen Commune each barefoot doctor treated an average of 1500 cases each year.[23] In Hunan Province a barefoot doctor was reported to have given over 14,000 treatments in a period somewhat longer than 3½ years.[24] A barefoot doctor called Li Hsunchao performed over 300 operations after 1967 in a commune in Kwangtung Province.[25] A young woman barefoot doctor in Hopei Province delivered 120 babies and gave 3700 acupuncture treatments during a period of just over two years.[26] Although it is difficult to determine what qualifies to be counted as a treatment, these figures certainly suggest that basic health care in China's countryside must be more extensive than any other developing country in Asia. In the communes which encircle Peking and are within the Peking administrative district there are over 12,000 barefoot doctors.[27] This figure is a good indicator of the success of the overall program because the peasants around Peking were traditionally among the very poorest in China.

The Instruction Manual for Barefoot Doctors

A great deal has been written on barefoot doctors in both China and the West, but it has been difficult to describe the scope of their work. It occurred to me as I looked over one of the few copies of *The Instruction Manual for Barefoot Doctors* in the United States that perhaps the best way to pin down the range of barefoot doctor work would be to survey the contents of the single book which each barefoot doctor has in his or her possession. To the best of my knowledge, no one in the West has yet written about this remarkable book.

First, a few words of introduction should be said about the book. It was edited by the Revolutionary Committee of Chiangchen Commune Hospital — the commune I have discussed so frequently in this essay. The editing was completed in January

1970, and the book was first published in June 1970 by the People's Medicine Publisher in Peking, and distributed by the New China Book Company. A total of 500,000 copies were printed in the first edition, the book contains 591 pages and almost half a million Chinese written characters, and the cost is 1 yuan (.40 ¢). There are, in fact, two different *Instruction Manuals for Barefoot Doctors* — one for use in north China, and one for use in south China. Although I have not yet seen the northern version, I assume it is basically the same in structure with the only differences being related to illnesses and treatments peculiar to conditions in north China.

The book begins with three articles about the development of the barefoot doctor program in Chiangchen Commune. The first of these was originally printed in both *Red Flag* magazine and the *People's Daily* of Peking; the second article was originally published in the Shanghai paper *Wen Hui Pao;* and the last article appears only in the *Instruction Manual.* These three pieces are important for barefoot doctors in the rest of south China because they describe precisely how barefoot doctors were recruited, trained, payed, and generally received in an area where the program is a success. Of course each of the articles places heavy emphasis on the political question of the need to concentrate on basic medical care for the peasant population, and stress preventive medicine while opposing careerism and over-specialization.

What follows is a brief outline of the major topics treated in the *Instruction Manual,* and a few of the specific diseases or illnesses discussed:

Chapter 1 Human Anatomy (4 pages)

Chapter 2 Prevention and Treatment of Common Diseases of the Respiratory Tract (30 pages) (influenza, bronchitis, asthma, emphysema, pneumonia, etc.)

Chapter 3 Prevention and Treatment of Common Diseases of the Digestive System (32 pages) (enterogastritis, ulcers, sclerosis of the liver, etc.)

Chapter 4 Prevention and Treatment of Common Parasitic and Communicable Diseases (76 pages) (malaria, schistosomiasis, measles, diphtheria, tuberculosis, meningitis, dysentery, typhoid, etc.)

Chapter 5   Prevention and Treatment of Common Diseases of Blood and the Circulatory System (45 pages) (rheumatic fever, anemia, etc.)

Chapter 6   Prevention and Treatment of Common Diseases of the Urinary Tract (12 pages) (kidney infection, kidney stone, etc.)

Chapter 7   Prevention and Treatment of Common Diseases of the Nervous System (18 pages) (epilepsy, hyperthyroidism, etc.)

Chapter 8   Prevention and Treatment of Common Disorders of the Skin, Bones, and Muscles (33 pages) (staph infection, acute acne, elephantiasis, mammitis, tetanus, hemorrhoids, arthritis, rheumatism, etc.)

Chapter 9   Prevention and Treatment with Regard to Birth Control and Gynecology (58 pages) (contraceptives, abortion, sterilization, childbirth complications, miscarriage, etc.)

Chapter 10   Prevention and Treatment of Common Diseases of Eyes, Ears, Nose, and Skin (22 pages) (tracoma, cataracts, etc.)

Chapter 11   Information about Prevention and Care of Tumors and Cancerous Growths (4 pages)

Chapter 12   Emergency Treatments and Poisoning (37 pages)

Chapter 13   Diagnosis and Treatment of Common Maladies which Occur Suddenly (13 pages) (high fever, convulsions, shock, coma, etc.)

Chapter 14   Rescue, and Treatment of Battle Wounds (21 pages) (bullet wounds, splinting, transportation of wounded, etc.)

Chapter 15   Common Chinese Herbal Medicines (131 pages) (207 herbs are discussed under such broad categories as cough prevention, fever reducing, heat prostration, laxatives, rheumatism, chills, congestion, blood treatments, diarrhea, digestion, vomitting, nutritious medicine, tranquilizers, preventing parasites, skin diseases)

Chapter 16   Methods of New Acupuncture (30 pages) (basic principles, common acupuncture points, new acupuncture treatments for common illnesses)

Charts
1) common medicines
2) norms for diagnosis
3) mixing medicines
4) tests for allergies (penicillin)
5) tests for poison allergies (anti-toxin)
6) antibiotics
7) standard weights and measures, and conversion tables
8) medicine dosage for children by age and weight

The layout of each section consists of various illustrations and diagrams related to the specific part of the body discussed, a list of symptoms to assist the barefoot doctor in making accurate diagnoses, and a variety of prescriptions and treatments for the specific illnesses. Each chapter generally includes a number of case studies for the reference of the barefoot doctor.[28]

The contents of the *Instruction Manual for Barefoot Doctors* reveal a number of interesting things. For example, included in the section on communicable and parasitic diseases is a full discussion of methods of eliminating insect pests such as mosquitoes which bear infectious diseases, methods of purifying water supplies and decontaminating human excreta which will be used as fertilizer, and methods of eliminating the fresh water snails which host the worm agent responsible for the schistosomiasis problem. In short, there is no distinction made between the importance of preventive techniques; and the actual practice of medicine itself. In fact, for China it can be argued that preventive medicine is far more important.

Secondly, there is great evidence of integrating traditional Chinese medicine and practice (herbal medicine and acupuncture) with modern Western practices (vaccinations and antibiotics). Barefoot doctors seem to learn very early how to give injections under sanitary conditions. Also, it is no coincidence that the largest section in the book is devoted to cataloging herbal medicines. Sketches of the herbs are provided to assist the barefoot doctors in locating the plants, and a description is offered of the probable location and growing season of the herbs. Further, the barefoot doctors are told how to prepare and mix the herbs, and under what conditions to prescribe the medicine. The various documents published on barefoot doctors since the term was first used in 1968 emphasize the need of barefoot doctors to seek out the traditional Chinese doctors who specialize in herbal medicine. A barefoot doctor of the Chuang nationality in Kwangsi Province, for example, travelled a total of 2000 kilometers to collect and record 1100 folk prescriptions, and 1800 separate herbs.[29] Most barefoot doctors seem to be able to prescribe between 200 and 300 prescriptions. Most barefoot doctors also seem to be able to master the application of acupuncture treatment for approximately 100 basic points of the body. It is also interesting to note that, aside from herbal medicines, the sections in the book which receive the most attention are those dealing with parasitic and communicable diseases, and birth control and childbirth.

Of course there is no reason to believe that all barefoot doctors are experienced enough to treat all the medical problems described in the *Instruction Manual*. Some are relatively advanced, and some are only beginners. I suspect that most barefoot doctors fall somewhere in between, and the longer they serve as barefoot doctors the more skilled they become. The documents published on the barefoot doctors since 1968 confirm the fact that barefoot doctors in various parts of China are in fact treating successfully many of the common but serious diseases and illnesses discussed in the *Instruction Manual*. What follows is a brief list of cases treated by barefoot doctors and subsequently mentioned in official documents published in China: rheumatism, influenza, hepatitis, hernia, cataracts, lymphatic tuberculosis, infantile paralysis, facial paralysis, optic atrophy, glaucoma, hypertension, neurasthenia, mastitis, diarrhea, measles, malaria, pneumonia, gastric ulcers, neuralgia, icterogenic spirochetosis, tonsillitis, sun-stroke, osteomyelitis, abcess of the foot, malnutrition due to indigestion, and deafness. Unhappily the documents do not report the failures which barefoot doctors most certainly have experienced.

CONCLUSION

The barefoot doctor program, since its inception in 1965, seems to be making tremendous strides in precisely the areas of greatest concern to China's peasantry. Wisely, the program concentrates most on the techniques of preventive medicine, but perhaps more important, it has raised political questions about the orientation of China's medical and health program. Medical personnel should be recruited from the countryside, and return to practice in the countryside. Each training course should be brief, and followed by practical work. Each successive training course should offer more advanced and specialized training, but no student should be tied down to classroom study for years at a time. Barefoot doctors should live among the people, work alongside them in the fields, and earn the same amount of money. Emphasis should be placed on diseases and illnesses common to the area where the barefoot doctor practices, and over-specialization should be discouraged. Finally, traditional Chinese herbal medicine and acupuncture should be the object of scientific analysis and practiced in conjunction with modern Western medicine. The implications of this type of program for Third World nations are quite obvious. It should not be surprising that the copy of the *Instruction Manual* which I used to prepare this study was not obtained in China, but rather in northern Burma. There is also much that physicians and medical workers in America and other industrially advanced countries can learn from the barefoot doctor approach. Why has general practice virtually disappeared from the American medical scene? Why the emphasis on specialization? Why are nurses and other medical workers restricted in their work, yet unable to enter medical school to obtain an M.D. degree? Why is the process of medical school, internship, and residency so long? Why is medical and health care so incredibly expensive? Whose interests are served by such powerful lobbies as the American Medical Association? In China all these sorts of problems would be raised as political questions.

FOOTNOTES

[1]For an overview of medical and health practice in China today see *China,*

Inside the People's Republic, New York: Bantam Press, 1972, Chapter 8 "Medicine," pp. 228-246.

[2] Joshua Horn, *Away With All Pests: An English Surgeon in People's China: 1954-69,* New York: Monthly Review Press, 1971, p. 125.

[3] Edgar Snow, *Red China Today, The Other Side of the River,* New York: Vintage Books, 1970, p. 75.

[4] *Ch'ih-chiao i-sheng p'ei-hsun-chiao-ts'ai* (Instruction Manual for Barefoot Doctors), Shanghai: People's Medicine Publisher, 1970. I want to thank Charles Martin of Harvard University for lending me his copy of the *Instruction Manual* (hereafter cited as IMBD).

[5] Horn, p. 125.

[6] Mao Tse-tung, "The United Front in Cultural Work," *Selected Works,* Vol. III, Peking: Foreign Language Press, p. 235.

[7] Mao Tse-tung, "In Memory of Norman Bethune," *Selected Works,* Vol. II, Peking: Foreign Language Press, p. 337.

[8] The statistics and information on Hungchiao Commune were gathered during my visit to that commune in June 1971; the statistics and information on Chiangchen Commune are in the IMBD, pp. 1-24.

[9] IMBD, 1-2.

[10] IMBD, 1. Writing in 1969 Joshua Horn uses the term "peasant doctors."

[11] IMBD, 18.

[12] New China News Agency (NCNA), "Ranks of Barefoot Doctors Grow Rapidly in Shanghai Area," October 10, 1969.

[13] IMBD, 3.

[14] NCNA, "An Outstanding Barefoot Doctor in Southwest China Border Province," June 26, 1970.

[15] IMBD, 2.

[16] IMBD, 2.

[17] IMBD, 2-3.

[18] IMBD, 7.

[19] IMBD, 6.

[20] NCNA, "A Medical School for Barefoot Doctors," April 18, 1969; NCNA, "Popular Rural Medical School in Northwest China," October 20, 1971.

[21] IMBD, 6.

[22] IMBD, 6.

[23] IMBD, 5.

[24] NCNA, "Shop Assistant Becomes Sparetime Barefoot Doctor," May 31, 1969.

[25] NCNA, "A Barefoot Doctor Serves Poor and Lower-Middle Peasants Wholeheartedly," July 8, 1969.

[26] NCNA, "Young Barefoot Doctor Welcomed by Poor and Lower-Middle Peasants in Tientsin, North China," March 17, 1970.

[27] NCNA, "Barefoot Doctors on Outskirts of Peking Mature Under Guidance of Chairman Mao's Revolutionary Line," Nov. 19, 1970.

[28] I would like to thank Helena Huang for helping me to identify the correct English translations for difficult Chinese medical terms.

[29] NCNA, "Outstanding Barefoot Doctor in South China Serves People Wholeheartedly," June 25, 1970.

Chapter 13

HEALTH CARE IN MODERN CHINA: AN EYEWITNESS REPORT

Samuel Rosen

OUR HISTORICAL AND MOST EXCITING JOURNEY began on September 14, 1971 when my wife and I left the train which had brought us from Hong Kong and walked over the border of the People's Republic of China. There, we were met by a pair of public health officials and, after lunch, led to another train ready for the trip to Canton. After a comfortable ride to the sounds of the Internationale which was booming from the train's loud speakers, we were greeted by Prof. Wu, head of otolarynogology, and a group of local physicians. They were accompanied by Mr. Chung, from Peking, a representative of the Chinese Medical Association which had invited us to visit China.

After Drs. Paul Dudley White and Grey Dimond arrived the next day with their wives, we began a tour of the nearby hospitals, schools, communes and factories. Our first choice was to visit a Chinese commune since nearly 600 million live in rural areas. The first commune was located about 30 miles north of Canton. Called Sing-Wa, it had a population of 61,000 divided into sixty-four cooperatives, each subdivided into 20 brigades and 326 production teams.

The commune we were privileged to see was a typical representative of the new rural organizations in the People's Republic of China. Its principal products were rice and vegetables while others near Hang-Chow, for example, mainly grew tea. The commune had at its disposal 5000 acres of arable land, and also raised hemp, cotton and fish. Part-time working housewives

147

and retired laborers added to their own income and that of the commune by engaging in a variety of communal enterprises, such as making noodles.

We were received by the chairman of the commune and the members of his executive committee together with the physician in charge of the local commune hospital. During our conversation these men and women told us about the conditions in that area before 1949 when a thousand people had to leave each year because they were starving to death. Lack of clothing, education and extreme poverty forced them to go to the urban centers to beg, or the landlord would take their children in payment for tax money.

The problem of water, either prolonged droughts or destructive floods, had been a chronic problem until recently. The commune has now built three reservoirs and is in the process of erecting another for the irrigation of the fields. Interestingly, the Chinese use a novel round rubber dam which can be inflated or emptied of water according to the water requirements. We were told that the commune had also established thirty power stations which furnished electricity for the irrigation schemes as well as light for the individual dwellings.

As a result of the technological advances, the members of the commune now raise more than they need to adequately feed their people. Consequently, the excess produce is sold to the government and the funds obtained are invested in machinery, trucks, clothing and bicycles.

Of primary importance to us was the health care set-up of this commune which was typical of other similar rural organizations in the country. At present, the main goal of the Chinese is the prevention of disease and the possibility of reaching and serving every man, woman and child of the People's Republic. Frequent meetings are held for the teaching of good hygienic practices to the participating peasants. The members of every commune spray DDT to eliminate mosquitoes, flies and bedbugs, and they trap rats with the result that these four time-honored pests have been practically eliminated.

In addition, the peasants have engaged in a vigorous campaign to eliminate schistosomiasis, a severe parasitic disease, by catching the intermediary host, the snails, which inhabit the waterways. For this purpose, they glide along the shores in small boats and bucket out the mud where the snails thrive, or they overturn the muddy border so deeply that the snails are buried. We were told that this work was carried out wherever symptoms and signs of schistosomiasis appeared. The campaigns of the last decade have virtually eliminated the disease and removed it from the list of endemic diseases in China.

With better hygiene and sanitary conditions, the infant mortality has been reduced by more than 90 percent since 1949. Women "barefoot doctors" are also trained as midwives in order that they can competently attend the women in labor. If any problem is foreseen or arises, the mother-to-be is taken to a hospital instead of giving birth at home.

The decrease in infant mortality has made birth control a highly desirable activity. The Chinese women use mainly the pill or a cervical ring and receive birth control information from the "barefoot doctors" or trained housewives. Although the emphasis is on methods of preventing conception, abortions can also be carried out when needed.

At the commune's hospital, the young Chinese surgeon explained to us the scope of his activities. The hospital had been built in 1958 but even as late as 1962 medical care had not been well organized. However, the hospital now had a staff of sixty-five health workers and had expanded its facilities to accommodate clinics, as well as maternity and otolaryngology wards. Before 1949, there were only 200 beds in this municipal hospital, while the present stucco building could accommodate 700 beds of which 340 were surgical and 80 assigned to pediatric patients. According to our host's account, he had performed over 400 surgical operations in the last two years without a case of wound infection. The hospital, which has radiological equipment, microscopes, and a laboratory with photocolorimeter, boasts a death rate of only 4 per thousand. Its staff carried out yearly a careful examination — including blood tests and x-rays — of every member of the commune who was checked for eleven important disease entities. The surgeon claimed to have performed delicate surgery in the commune's hospital: he reconstructed the hand of a man who had accidentally suffered the amputation of four fingers, and repaired the club foot of a young girl.

Although the hospital does not have any chemist on its staff, there exists a pharmaceutical laboratory for the preparation of traditional Chinese herbs for medical purposes. Many of the herbs are raised right outside the hospital and collected by health workers who transform them into extracts sealed into sterile ampules. For thousands of years the Chinese have gathered herbs from the fields, roamed forests and climbed mountains in order to discover plants with medicinal value. Today, the government of the People's Republic encourages the development of traditional medicines side by side with the elaboration of modern "Western" medicines in the belief that both can be valuable and useful to the patient. When we consider the value of Rauwolfia, ephedrin and the opiates in our therapeutical armamentarium, it is not difficult to understand the respect which the Chinese accord to traditional herbs.

If the rural setting suggested a certain lack of sophistication in the practice of medicine, this impression was quickly dispelled. We were all sitting around a table discussing coronary heart disease when the medical director — barely 42 years old — declared that he suffered from a coronary occlusion two years ago. Being renowned cardiologists, Drs. White and Grey Dimond got very excited and demanded to see the physician's clinical record. Sure enough, the director came back with a lengthy dossier containing all the results of laboratory examinations currently carried out in the West.

At the brigade level, there was a smaller health station manned by a so-called "barefoot doctor" and a few peasant health workers. The brigade takes care of 605 households or 2700 people unless the more serious nature of the medical problem suggests a transfer to the commune's hospital. All the people are taught hygienic principles and their children receive the basic immunizations against tetanus, typhoid, diphtheria and whooping cough. They also receive smallpox and the B.C.G. or anti-tuberculosis vaccine. Children are checked more often than adults, and careful records are kept concerning the vaccination schedules.

The training of a "barefoot doctor" varies considerably.

Usually, they spend three to six months at a hospital where they are given a basic course of training in anatomy, diagnosis, acupuncture, simple therapeutics and other skills such as injection techniques. The "barefoot doctors" work closely with a medical doctor in the commune, and they often meet together to discuss their patients and medical problems. Thus, such a contact can well be considered as a process of continuing education and acquisition of practical experience for the "barefoot doctor."

While we were visiting the health station, I glanced at the "barefoot doctor's" desk where East and West symbolically met. Here was an acupuncture mannikin with its hundreds of points and related meridians, a nest of acupuncture needles immersed in alcohol, together with a stethoscope, a blood pressure apparatus and books containing the quotations of Chairman Mao.

I decided that I would like to know just how a procedure such as acupuncture would feel and prevailed upon the "barefoot doctor" to demonstrate it on me. After examining my blood pressure and heart sounds, he consented. I sat down in a rather comfortable chair, pulled up my trouser leg, while Drs. Dimond and White with their wives and my wife hovered over me with a combination of concern and photographic cameras. The young "barefoot doctor" and his co-worker carefully sterilized with alcohol a spot just below both knees and just above both wrists, and then proceeded to insert some fine and flexible needles about 2 cm. deep into the skin. I felt nothing except for a small wave of heat as the Chinese twirled the inserted needles and then quickly withdrew them.

From the above it is obvious that in China there exists a network of medical care extending from the field through the brigade health center all the way to the commune's hospital. The latter even sends out mobile units to the countryside to work with the peasants and teach the "barefoot doctors."

We also had occasion to visit the Capital Hospital, probably one of the largest institutions in Peking. Not only did the hospital boast a large outpatient department, maternity ward and pediatric as well as otolaryngology patients, but it possessed a fine medical library with the latest journals from all over the world. Here Dr. White saw a copy of the *New England Journal of Medicine* barely three months old, while Dr. Dimond was shown the *Kansas State Medical Journal* and I was handed the *Journal of the Mt. Sinai Hospital of New York,* a kind gesture of the gracious Chinese hosts to their foreign guests.

I would like to conclude with some impressions concerning my own medical specialty: the treatment of the deaf. We went to visit schools for the deaf in three major urban centers: Peking, Canton and Shanghai. These children had been gathered from the surrounding villages in 1968 and placed in schools where they were trained phonetically, just as we do. They were either living at the school or being bused-in.

In all the three schools which we visited the training was excellent. The children were taught how to dance — some tried ballet — and to play musical instruments without the use of hearing aids. All the children we observed had nerve deafness which is mostly of a congenital nature. The acupuncture treatment employed varied considerably. Although the "barefoot doctors" carefully explain the treatment to the children, it is not a painless thing. However, the patients are stoic and never move even a muscle although I could tell that it was hurting.

We were in China 32 days but never once did we hear a child cry. Those in charge of the treatments reported that the children were improving, but I had no idea what the children's hearing was like before they entered the school. Moreover, I had no time to test their hearing at the time of my visits — even if I had done so the lack of any data to compare with would have made the whole trip useless. The Chinese declare that these acupuncture treatments are new and still in the experimental stage, thus their validity and usefulness is still in question.

I was very curious to see a stapes mobilization procedure in the People's Republic of China, and had the opportunity of doing so in Shanghai. A young surgeon, Dr. Chow, was scheduled to operate on a forty-two year old woman who had had a successful operation in the other ear two years prior. To my delight, I watched my Chinese counterpart operate on the second ear step by step through a monocular microscope of six magnifications which he had constructed by himself. His work was as fine as I have seen performed anywhere in the world, and this was characteristic of Chinese medical and surgical practice everywhere we went.

Instead of looking down condescendingly on the Chinese, we would do well to remember that theirs is an ancient civilization going back uninterruptedly for more than five millenia. However, I think that what impressed me most in China was the devotion of their medical men and women to the primary goal set by them and for them in society: to bring medicine to the people. In essence this means furnishing preventive and medical care to almost a quarter of the human race, a gigantic undertaking by all standards. Following my visit, I believe that the Chinese are suceeding to a remarkable degree in doing just that.

PART V
(CONCLUSION AND BIBLIOGRAPHY)

(CONCLUSION)

Guenter B. Risse

SINCE OUR MEETING WAS HELD last April there have been a series of favorable developments in the United States regarding acupuncture and traditional Chinese medicine. At some medical centers there are now plans to carry out small clinical research projects concerning the analgesic qualities of acupuncture and how this method compares with our conventional analgesic drugs.

Another reflection of the growing interest is the creation of committees to investigate the potential use of acupuncture in the U.S. and study the legal barriers it faces. The California Medical Association has already established such a formal mechanism to gather information and eventually promulgate new guidelines.

More recently, an invitation extended to a group of prominent Chinese physicians to visit the U.S. has been accepted. Conversely, the Chinese have invited a delegation of academic physicians from the University of California in Los Angeles to visit the mainland later this year. Thus, further contacts between the medical personnel of both countries seem to be in the offing, a decisive factor for our understanding of Chinese acupuncture and health care delivery.

In the meantime, continued caution, especially regarding the practice of acupuncture, is highly advisable. This attitude has been repeatedly expressed by the Chinese medical authorities such as Dr. Chang, the American trained director of Peking's Friendship Hospital where acupuncture anesthesia is used. Recently, the American Society of Anesthesiologists issued a press release expressing their grave concern over the premature application of acupuncture to American patients for relief of pain during surgery.

Although some procedures such as a skin graft and a tonsillectomy have apparently been performed with success, acupuncture anesthesia is still in its early experimental stages. Basic research into the neurophysiology of pain and clinical investigations of the methods and results obtained in operative and postoperative analgesia will in time provide answers to the rather puzzling questions being raised today. In the meantime let us not prematurely convert the entire United States, as Dr. Rosen asserts, into a giant pin-cushion!

REFERENCES

Liu, Wei-Chi: "Acupuncture anesthesia: a case report," *J.A.M.A.* 221 (1972), 87-88.

Press Release, The American Society of Anesthesiologists, June 2, 1972.

"Acupuncture intrigues physicians," *American Medical News* (June 19, 1972), 1 and 11.

"Pins against pain," *Time Newsmagazine,* (June 12, 1972), 44.

(BIBLIOGRAPHY)

The following is a short list of useful books and articles—some already cited in the various papers—about the topics covered during the Symposium. While it makes no pretense of being complete in any subject matter, the numerous titles are representative of the current literature available in our libraries and book stores. (Ed.)

1) General

Adams, Ruth, ed.: *Contemporary China,*
New York, Vintage Books, 1966

Committee of Concerned Asian Scholars, *China! Inside the People's Republic,*
New York, Bantam Books, 1972

Creel, Herrlee G.: *Chinese Thought from Confucius to Mao-Tse-tung,*
Chicago, Univ. of Chicago Press, 1953

de Bary, William T.: *Sources of Chinese Tradition,*
New York, Columbia Univ. Press, 1960

Myrdal, Jan: *Report from a Chinese Village*
Translation from Swedish by M. Michael,
New York, Pantheon Books, 1965

Myrdal, Jan and Kessle, Gun: *China: The Revolution Continued,*
Transl. from rev. Swedish ed. by P. Britten Austin,
New York, Pantheon Books, 1970

Needham, Joseph: *Science and Civilization in China,*
Vol. I "Introductory Orientations,"
Cambridge: Univ. Press, 1954
Vol. II "History of Scientific Thought,"
Cambridge, Univ. Press, 1956

Needham, Joseph: *Clerks and Craftsmen in China and the West,*
Cambridge, Univ. Press, 1970

Schram, Stuart R.: *Mao Tse-Tung,*
Baltimore, Penguin Books, 1966

Snow, Edgar: *Red China Today: the Other Side of the River,*
New York, Vintage Books, 1971

Thomson, James C., Jr.: *While China Faced West,*
Cambridge, Harvard Univ. Press, 1969

Tse-Tung, Mao: *Quotations from Chairman Mao Tse-Tung,*
Peking, Foreign Language Press, 1966

Yu-lan, Fung: *A History of Chinese Philosophy,*
Princeton, Princeton Univ. Press, 1952

II) *Ancient Chinese Medicine*

Chen, C. Y.: *History of Chinese Medical Science,*
Hong Kong, Chinese Med. Inst., 1968

Chen, Ronald: *The History and Method of Physical Diagnosis in
    Classical Chinese Medicine,*
New York, Vantage Press, 1969

Chang-Hui-Chien, *Li Shih-Chen — Great Pharmacologist of Ancient
    China,*
Peking: Foreign Languages Press, 1960

Huard, Pierre and Wong, Ming: *Chinese Medicine,*
transl. from the French by B. Fielding,
New York, McGraw-Hill, 1968

Lee, T., Ch'eng, C. F., and Chang, C. S.: "Some early records of
    nervous and mental diseases in traditional Chinese medicine,"
Chinese Med. J. 81 (1962), 55-59

Lee, T.: "Medical ethics in Ancient China,"
Bull. Hist. Med. 13 (1943), 268-277

Needham, J. and Lu, G. D.: "Chinese medicine," in F.N.L. Poynter,
    ed., *Medicine and Culture,*
London, Wellcome Inst. Hist. Med., 1969, pp. 255-314

Needham, J. and Lu, G. D.: "Records of diseases in Ancient China,"
    in D. Brothwell and A. T. Sandison, eds., *Diseases in Antiquity,*
Springfield, Thomas, 1967, pp. 222-237

Palos, Stephan: *The Chinese Art of Healing,*
New York, Herder and Herder, 1971

Veith, I.: "The supernatural in Far Eastern concepts of mental dis-
    ease," *Bull. Hist. Med.* 27 (1963), 139-158

Veith, Ilza (ed. & transl.): *Huang Ti Nei Ching Su Wên, the Yellow Emperor's Classic of Internal Medicine*, new ed.,
Berkeley, Univ. of California Press, 1966

Wallhöfer, Heinrich – Anna von Rottauscher, *Chinese Folk Medicine*,
New York, New American Library, 1972

Ware, James R. (ed. & transl.), *Alchemy, Medicine, and Religion in the China of A.D. 320: the Nei P'ien of Ko Hung,*
Cambridge, M.I.T. Press, 1966

III) *Chinese Acupuncture*

Dimond, E. G.: "Acupuncture anesthesia, Western medicine and Chinese traditional medicine," *J.A.M.A.* 218 (1971), 1558-1563

Dufour, Roger: *Atlas d' Acupuncture Topographique en Vingt-trois Regions,*
Paris, Le François, 1960

Duke, Marc: *Acupuncture,*
New York, Pyramid House, 1972

Lavier, Jacques: *Points of Chinese Acupuncture*, transl. from French by P. Chancellor,
Rustington, England, Health Science Press, 1965

Mann, Felix: *Acupuncture: the Ancient Chinese Art of Healing,*
New York, Vintage Books, 1972

Mann, Felix: *The Meridians of Acupuncture,*
London, Heinemann, 1964

Peking Academy of Traditional Chinese Medicine, *Chinese Therapeutical Methods of Acupuncture and Moxibustion,*
Peking, Foreign Languages Press, 1960

Stiefvater, Erich W.: *Akupunktur als Neuraltherapie*, 2. ed.,
Ulm, Haug, 1956

Veith, I.: "Acupuncture therapy – past and present," *J.A.M.A.* 180 (1962), 478-484

IV) *Modern Chinese Medicine*

Balme, Harold: *China and Modern Medicine,*
London, London Missionary Soc., 1921

Bowers, J. Z.: "The founding of Peking Union Medical College: policies and personalities," *Bull. Hist. Med.* 45 (1971), 305-321

Croizier, Ralph C.: *Traditional Medicine in Modern China,*
Cambridge, Harvard Univ. Press, 1968

Farber, Knud: *Report on Medical Schools in China,*
Geneva, League of Nations Health Organization, 1931

Ferguson, Mary E.: *China Medical Board and Peking Union Medical College: a Chronicle of Fruitful Collaboration 1914-1951,*
New York, China Med. Bd. of N.Y., 1970

Horn, Joshua S.: *Away with All Pests: an English Surgeon in People's China 1954-1969,*
New York and London, Monthly Review Press, 1969

Hume, Edward H.: *Doctors East, Doctors West, an American Physician's Life in China,*
New York, Norton, 1946

Koran, L. M.: "Psychiatry in Mainland China: history and recent status," *Amer. J. Psychiatry* 128 (1972), 970-977

Orleans, L. A.: *Medical Education and Manpower in Communist China,* ed. by C. T. Hu,
New York, Teachers' College Press, Columbia Univ., 1969

Worth, R. M.: "Health trends in China since the Great Leap Forward," *China Quarterly* 22 (1965), 181-189

INDEX

A

Abortions, 113, 142, 149
Acupuncture, 13, 26-28, 40, 41, 44-45, 49-95, 108, 138, 143, 144, 145
  concern over premature application, 52-53, 157-158
  definition, 49
  effects, 60
  electro-acupuncture, 40, 53-54, 65, 69-71, 89-90, 93-94
  history 26, 50
  in Japan, 28
  mechanisms, 72-74, 81
  needles, 26, 50, 56, 65, 71, 72
  neurophysiological bases for, 72-74, 85-87, 89-95
  origins, 49-50
  points, 26, 50, 58-61, 71, 82, 83
  psychological factors, 54, 62, 65, 71, 79, 87, 88, 90
  rationale, 26, 27, 50-52
  "stimulation quantity," 81-85, 88
  technique, 26, 53, 56-62, 65, 71, 77-80, 82-83
  theory, 45, 51-52, 67, 72-74, 81-87
  treatment for deafness, 152
  types of operations, 71
  veterinary applications, 68
Acupuncture anesthesia (analgesia), 53-55, 64-68, 69-75, 81-88, 107
  goiter surgery, 64
  lung removal, 77-80
  mechanisms, 81
  neurophysiological bases for, 72-74, 85-87, 89-95
  origins, 53, 70, 85
  problems, 54, 64-65, 83
  requirements. 61-62, 71-72
  statistics, 67, 75

  techniques, 61-62, 82-83
  theory, 72-74, 81, 85-87
  types of operations, 71
Anatomy, 18, 19, 45
  ancestor veneration, 18
  five Tsang, 19
  six Fu, 19
Anesthesia (conventional), 64-66, 74, 78, 80

B

Barefoot doctors, 43-45, 100, 116, 118-121, 125-145, 150-152
  origins, 132-133
  salaries, 121, 135
  training, 118, 119, 129, 130-132, 136-138, 150-151
  treatments, 138, 140, 144
  women, 113, 134, 135, 149
Bethune, Norman, 114, 128-129
Bioelectric currents, 85-87
Birth control, 45, 112-113, 142, 144, 149
Breathing, importance of in acupuncture, 62, 72, 79, 88

C

Careerism, 40, 41, 134-135, 139, 141, 145
Cauterization, 51
Chang Tsung-liang, 32, 33
Ch'en Kuo-fu, 35, 37
Ch'i (vital force), 50, 62, 70, 82, 88
Ch'i Po, 14, 15, 21, 27
Chiangchen Commune, 130-141
China
  Ministry of Health, 34, 37, 39

163